HEALTHY ME
HEALTHY WE

THE PATHWAY TO REALATIONSHIPS

BY DR. CHARLES FRAZIER, CHERYL GRAYSON, WILBUR PIKE III

FOREWORD BY DR. JOHN SCHERER

Copyright © 2025 by Charles Frazier, Cheryl Grayson, and Wilbur Pike III

All rights reserved.

No part of this publication may be reproduced, distributed, or transmitted in any form or by any means, including photocopying, recording, or other electronic or mechanical methods, without the prior written permission of the publisher, except as permitted by U.S. copyright law.

For permission requests, contact Charles Frazier at charles@ris-ct.com.

The stories, all names, characters, and incidents portrayed in this publication are fictitious. No identification with actual persons (living or deceased), places, buildings, and products are intended or should be inferred.

The authors have made every effort to ensure the accuracy of the information within this book was correct at time of publication. The authors take no responsibility for any loss, damage, or disruption caused by errors or omissions, whether such errors or omissions result from accident, negligence, or any other cause.

Book Cover by G. Logan Vega

Illustrations by G. Logan Vega and Cheryl Grayson

First published 2025

Printed in the United States of America

Library of Congress Cataloging-in-Publication Data Healthy Me, Healthy We The Pathway To REALationships / written by Charles Frazier, Cheryl Grayson, and Wilbur Pike III / edited by Natalie Schriefer / cover design and graphics by G. Logan Vega and Cheryl Grayson / interior layout by G. Logan Vega

ISBN 979-8-218-58516-7

1. Relationships – Development 2. Self – Help 3. Therapy/Counseling 4. Self-Empowerment 5. Individual Development –Creative stories 6. Personal Effectiveness

HEALTHY ME HEALTHY WE

The Pathway to REALationships

BY DR. CHARLES FRAZIER, CHERYL GRAYSON,
WILBUR PIKE III

FOREWORD BY DR. JOHN SCHERER

TABLE OF CONTENTS

I. Dedication

II. Preface

VI. Acknowledgements

VII. Foreword

Preparing to Embark..................pg.14

Deck 1 - Explore Deck................pg.53

Deck 2 - Accept & Heal Deck..........pg.90

Deck 3 - Grow Deck... ....pg.128

Deck 4 - Authentic Self Deck........pg.149

Deck 5 - Share Deck...................pg.190

Deck 6 - Align Deck..................pg. 216

Deck 7 - Pursue Deck.................pg. 235

Deck 8 - Commit Deck.................pg. 265

Deck 9 - Fortify Deck................pg. 293

From the Bridge......................pg. 319

Dedication

This workbook is dedicated to everyone who has ever wondered, **"What can I do to make things better?"**

This question contains the one word that indicates a sincere desire for healthier interactions, hook-ups, and interpersonal outcomes...that word being **"I."**

To start with **SELF** in improving relationships is the core tenet of this workbook. May you be compelled to share your learnings with those closest to you so that, by extension, we'll all help one another as we grow stronger and healthier.

"Wishing you healthy interactions and interpersonal outcomes,
- Charles, Cheryl, and Wilbur"

Preface

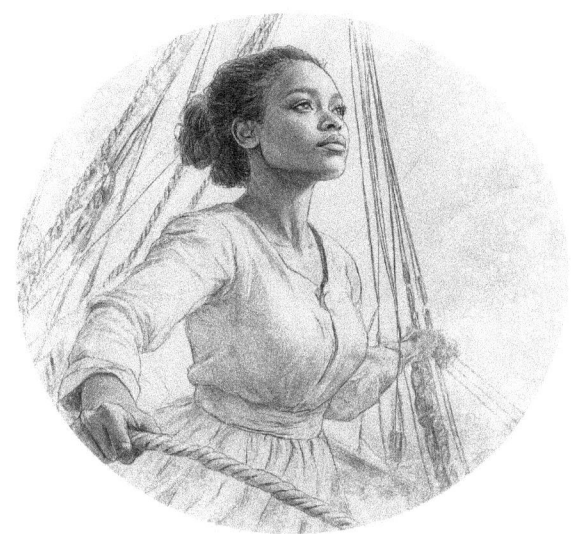

"You cannot control the wind, but you can adjust your sails."

~ *African Proverb*

Have you ever felt like a passenger on the Titanic? Scared, sad, confused, maybe even hopeless? During those situations, have you felt the need to send out a distress signal, but were unsure where to send it? If you were successful in sending your S.O.S., did you get the right kind of help?

Whether or not we recognize and acknowledge it, life is a journey. We've all felt disoriented, depressed, overwhelmed, and alone at times. This workbook was created as a tool to help you navigate the inevitable rough winds and choppy waters of life. In this book, you'll find examples and terms related to travel by sea. With that awareness and understanding, we provide approaches for managing common currents in a healthy way. As you continue on your voyage, it will be beneficial for you to think about the type of vessel you connect with most.

Do you relate to a big, beautiful cruise ship? Or how about a commercial tug boat, slow and cumbersome, but vital to help larger vessels reach their moorings? Do you connect best with a sleek sailboat, moving with and maximizing the wind? Perhaps you align best with the look and feel of a private motor yacht, expensive but beautiful, demonstrating your success in life.

All vessels have a set of assets and liabilities. Your goal is to maximize your assets and manage your liabilities. The first step in that process is to learn all you can about how your vessel works.

You'll read stories about how others have dealt with storms and difficult passages. You'll likely recognize similarities between their situations and yours while also getting an opportunity to imagine how you'd handle such situations. This will help you emerge with an enhanced understanding of how effectively you're functioning on your specific journey. Overall, you'll be better prepared to connect with others more authentically and, as a result, in a healthier manner.

Although we provide suggestions in these pages, keep in mind that no one's life is all smooth sailing and fair weather! In fact, ask any sailor, and they'll admit there are moments when they've had no control over the waters they're navigating. Realize instead that our goal is to help guide you to achieve healthier relationships, first with knowledge of yourself, and then with others.

Here is an important mindset to maintain as you work through this book: "Healthy Me, Healthy We " is a model to discover, understand, accept, and respect yourself—warts and all, the authentic YOU. The model represents what you know about yourself and how that authentic knowing helps to keep your voyage on the right course for YOU. In the process of connecting with yourself, you may find forgotten/sunken treasures along with past hurts. Though this can be difficult, it's also necessary, because it leads to gaining clarity, comfort, and confidence with yourself, which is critical for navigating your journey and applying the right tools to establish healthy relationships. This book is a practical guide for those who want to stop running from their truths and start working on themselves, from the inside out.

To that end, we'll help you to examine all the "ships" in your marina: friendships, companionships, intimate partnerships, and situation-ships. Each of these requires a variety of tools. For a healthy journey, we must also dismantle the misinformation we have relied upon since childhood, such as the old adage, "If we just do everything right at the right time, everything will turn out right." Said another way, we must accept the fact that, like those sailors mentioned earlier, we will discover facts and encounter situations over which we have no control. It doesn't mean we are powerless, but rather that we must acknowledge and develop our personal capabilities and apply them effectively when required.

The authors of this book are fellow voyagers. We are a part of your growth process, but with information and experience gained from our educations, backgrounds, and professions as clinicians and life coaches, respectively. We provide this information because we believe there is a healthier way to engage in the journey of life. Our mission is to help our readers better understand both their personal journey and how to use it to create healthier relationships with others.

This book is to help you find You, be You, and bring You—to all your relationships.

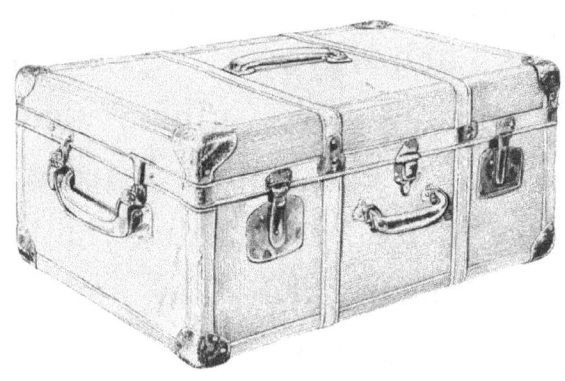

Acknowledgements

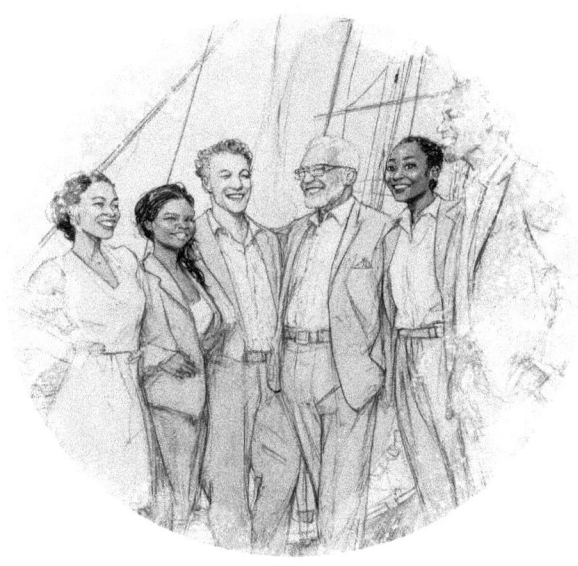

To all the individuals we've had the honor to counsel, coach, or train, we thank you for sharing your experiences and providing validity for the **Healthy Me, Healthy We** model. We thank John Scherer for writing the foreword as his work regarding individual breakthroughs and workplace transformations has inspired us. We see our work as part of the plethora of resources available to help people become their best selves and to connect with others in a healthy manner.

A very special "thank-you" goes to our editor, Natalie Schriefer whose exceptional skills helped to eliminate the errors and clarify the critical! To that end, our words would be far less appealing were it not for our extremely talented layout artist, Logan Vega. Logan's passion for rendering each page an elegant masterpiece that intersects art and words is peerless. Lastly, thank you to our families for giving us firsthand knowledge of the power of healthy, not perfect, relationships.

Foreword

Dr. John J. Scherer

***Everyone wants to have
healthy relationships.***

The challenge is practicing what it takes to create and sustain them. You, the reader, know this well.

Help has arrived: The authors of Healthy Me, Healthy We have given us a virtual handbook for how to have healthy relationships, and the first thing they want us to understand is that this challenge can best be seen as a life-long journey on a ship.

As a veteran of four years on a U.S. Navy Destroyer, I can attest to the accuracy of the many life-at-sea dimensions presented here. Regardless of the changing weather and the shifting state of the ocean—both things out of our control—we do our best to live and love and get meaningful work done, all of which happen in relationships. When thinking about how to get along with other people, the (human) "default" starting point is to focus on those other people and how they need to be different.

In case you haven't noticed, this doesn't work.

Fortunately, the authors have given us a unique, well-thought-out, simple-yet-profound approach to being "at sea" with other people, one that can help us "cruise" from where we are to where we want to be, by focusing first, not on others, but on ourselves. Great relationships begin with discovering who I am, who I really am, the authentic ME.

There is so much to like in this book, but one thing you will find especially helpful are the many practical, real-world-oriented exercises that introduce particularly useful skills or practices. As interesting as the principles taught here are, by far the most important intention of the authors is providing deep learning experiences that will impact your behavior, the way you ARE from moment-to-moment. By discovering and stepping fully into your own more Authentic Self, you are then in a position—and have earned the right—to create meaningful relationships with others. You can find many books about the need to be more authentic. Healthy Me, Healthy We actually shows us HOW.

> *"Being challenged in life is inevitable. Being defeated is optional."*
> ~Roger Crawford

This is one of many provocative quotes you will find here. This one encourages us to not give up on our journey when the weather is bad and the sea gets rough, but to continue to lean into our most challenging relationships, transforming them with the skills and practices laid out for us here.

In closing, I have been a gestalt therapist and a personal/leadership development coach for over 50 years, focusing on authenticity as THE key to effectiveness and fulfillment. In practicing the exercises the authors offer us here, I have learned even more about authenticity and about who I am. Practical wisdom. That's what is here for us all.
I am grateful for it.
I think you will be, too.

~Dr. John. J. Scherer

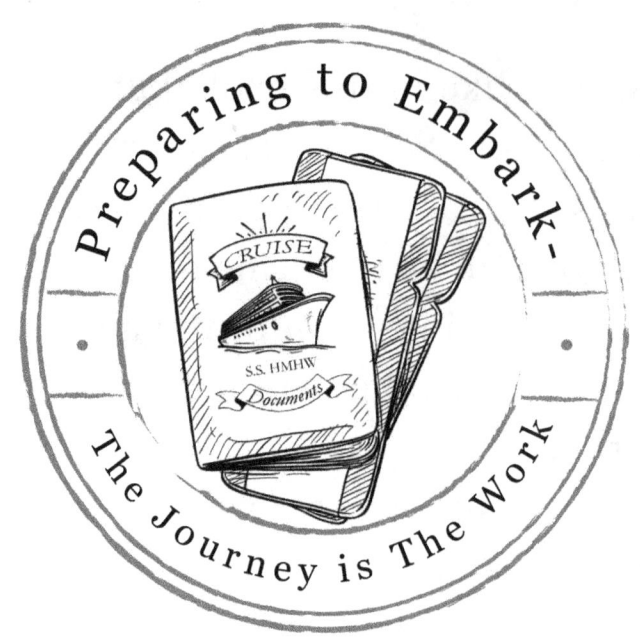

Preparing to Embark-
The Journey is The Work

CRUISE DOCUMENTS

Before joining us on this journey to healthy relationships, be sure to read your cruise documents—the information below will be a handy reference while you travel through this workbook.

As your crew, we provide these important concepts and activities as preparation for your journey, just like a real cruise. In the Cruise Documents, you'll learn that the goal of "Healthy Me, Healthy We" is Healthy and not Perfection.

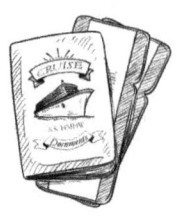

The cruise documents also allow you to:

- Take preliminary steps to stop running from yourself and start working on yourself.
- Recognize that the priority of your voyage is to seek, find, and understand your Authentic Self—not a partner, friend, or companion.
- Learn that being alone is not disastrous, but rather an opportunity to learn about yourself.
- Acknowledge that it's possible to be alone without feeling lonely.
- Explore the reality that there are no quick fixes for your issues, but that being REAL with yourself is the best path to being healthy.
- Realize that despite experiencing challenges in relationships, it is scientifically proven that people are wired to connect with others; we can use that knowledge to keep hope afloat.

BOOK LAYOUT & SECTIONS

To navigate the information in this book, we've established the following structure, which uses typical ship and/or cruise terms:

Preparing - *Cruise Documents:*

Information that is basic to understanding our approach, what's expected as you learn, and resources you may want to return to review or share with others.

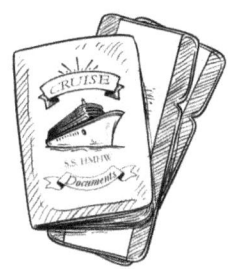

Decks - *Chapters*

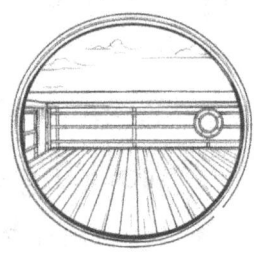

All good books are organized with chapters that hold related information. In this book, we call those the DECKS of the ship, and like when on a cruise, we've clustered related information into decks.

Charters - *Topics*

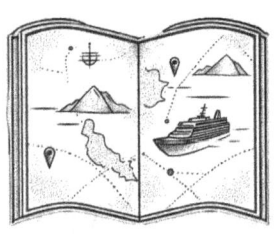

Some decks have more charters than others. Regardless of how many, charters indicate what can be learned/discovered on that deck. Charters take you to different areas of the deck.

Excursions - *Activities*

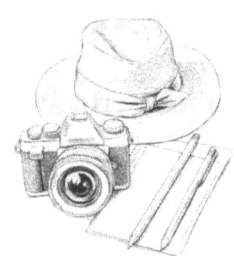

While on a deck and taking a charter, there are excursions or activities to help apply and reinforce concepts/information. We encourage you to take advantage of every excursion so that you can deepen your understanding!

Anchors - *Takeaways/High Points:*

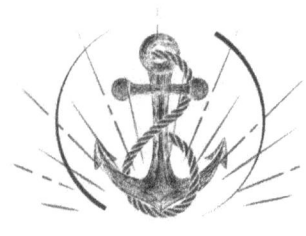

Think of the anchors as your souvenirs—what voyage would be complete without having something to remember it by? Share what you learn (and its impact on you) with others who may benefit from your learning and growth.

Healthy vs Perfection: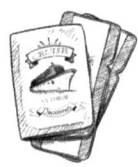

Utopia

/juːˈtoʊ.pi.ə/

"An imagined place or state of things in which everything is perfect."

We start with debunking the myth of "Happily Ever After," that familiar outcome of fairytales that inspires us mortals to seek similar results: A royal who sweeps us off our feet and whisks us off to a perfect life. A quick read of current headlines reveals that life doesn't even work that way for ACTUAL royals!

Someone once said that a perfect relationship cannot be achieved because once we enter the relationship it becomes *imperfect*. Although perfect relationships don't exist, healthy ones do. Having healthy relationships is like wearing suitable clothing: while the outfit may not be perfect, it still fits and looks good. To fit properly, the garment may need adjustments like hemming or tailoring for a *better fit*.

A healthy relationship is an *ongoing journey throughout which change is constant*. In addition to change being inevitable, it also invites some degree of conflict. For those reasons, we must realize that "healthy" means neither perfect nor conflict-free. To be "healthy" means that when conflict arises, we don't flee from it, fight it, or blame others.

Instead, we work through conflicts to resolve them and, thereby, strengthen our relationships. Conflicts present an opportunity to gain and apply better insights about yourself and others. Healthy individuals have learned how to work through difficult times without destroying themselves or others.

Healthy vs Perfection

Take a moment to think about your current or past relationships. [Tip: Focus on one type of relationship at a time—intimate, family, friends, etc.]

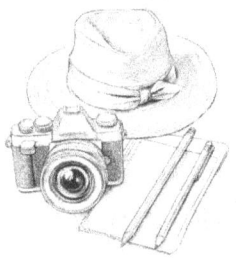

From the list below, circle the statements that you've experienced. After doing so for each type of relationship, determine if there are any patterns across relationships. As a final step, make a note of what was missing from those relationships; those "missing components" are opportunities for development/growth.

- Capacity to see good in each other
- Desire to do the right thing
- Demonstration of self-control
- Creating safe spaces to be your authentic selves
- Not panicking when conflict occurs
- Being available to learn
- Giving yourself (and others) permission to make mistakes
- Accepting your partner's perspective without trying to change it
- The goal is NOT to win but rather to understand the other person
- Love is a choice and not just a feeling

- Trust results from transparency and truth (T+T=T2)
- You (and your partner) can express yourselves without hostility

How to get healthier:

Like happiness, getting healthier is an inside job. It starts with you and your mindset, meaning your state of mind. Affirmations are one small way to adjust your mindset. You can start right now! The affirmations below can help you steady yourself on the journey to happiness. Try repeating them aloud when you're feeling stressed or overwhelmed:

- Though this journey focuses on me, I can and should enlist the help of trusted others.
- The final decisions about the direction and speed of my journey belong to me.
- Maintaining a "Healthy Me" is a continuous process and can only be navigated by me.
- I must look inside, own what I find, and accept responsibility for managing it.
- Each time I am tempted to point out another person's contribution to a problem, I will stop and ask myself, "Which dish did I bring to this potluck?"
- I will replace blaming thoughts with this one: The only person I can repair is me.
- I strive to bring the healthiest ME I can to my relationships, knowing that healthy doesn't mean perfect.

Anchors - *Takeaways*

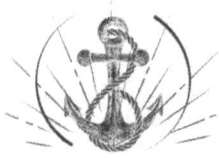

- There is no such thing as "…and they lived happily ever after."
- We should replace that fairytale ending with "…and they strove every day to be healthy individuals in healthy relationships."

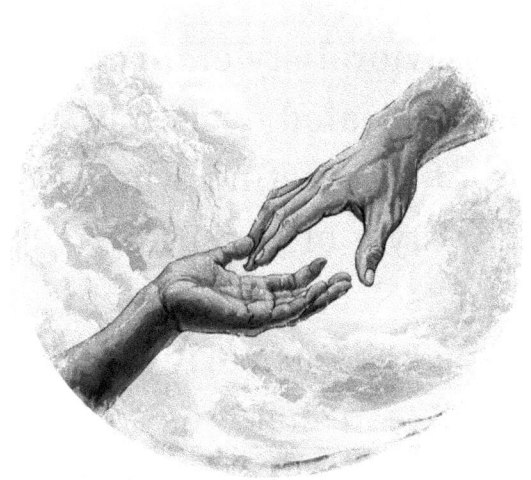

"People who need people are the luckiest people in the world."
~ *Styne/Merrill, Funny Girl, 1964*

What's in Everybody's Baggage?

Born for Human Connections (Attachment, Love, and Hate)

For psychological survival, humans require some degree of attachment to others. Yet despite that truth, there are interpersonal dynamics that can erode—or even prevent—healthy human connections. Furthermore, as children, the quality of our initial connections (with those on whom we rely to meet our basic needs for food, shelter, support) can shape our future relationship skills. For example, think about the child who, orphaned at a young age, must fend for him/herself. Such a tragedy can, indeed, reveal personality strengths of the child; the child will later rely upon this self-protective mental model to survive and get their needs met as an adult.

Each of us has a behavioral style: a collection of actions we engage in that, when repeated over time, form a pattern. For example, our style of interacting when we lead is called a leadership style; our style of parenting is called a parenting style. Our style of selecting, engaging in, and ending relationships is shaped by our early attachments; examining that behavioral style can help us gain awareness about vestiges of our personal past that prevent us from sustaining healthy relationships.

What does this mean in practical terms? That orphaned child may become an adult who struggles to connect with others; they may become lonely, distant, or angry. A child whose parent was unavailable may become overly dependent on others. This person may find it difficult to make decisions on their own and may sabotage relationships without realizing it by requiring constant reassurance.

Studies have proven that humans whose emotional connection to others has been eliminated or curtailed undergo unfathomable levels of stress— well beyond that created by hypertension, obesity, and smoking cigarettes!
In fact, studies have also shown that the opposite effect occurs for those with positive emotional connections, including accelerated recovery from potentially fatal illnesses like cancer. This understanding of the human need for connection is what underpins the solitary confinement practices of penal institutions—they use solitary confinement as a means of punishing inmates. On a smaller scale, this is the basis for the common parenting practice of "time-outs" for misbehaving toddlers.

No matter how you slice it, people need people. Despite instinctively needing one another, however, there is no guarantee that we instinctively know how best to sustain healthy connections with one another. That's where **this workbook comes in.**

> ### *Anchors* - *Takeaways*
>
>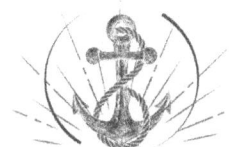
>
> - Healthy relationships make people stronger.
> - Connecting with others doesn't mean abandoning oneself.

Guiding Lights: Searching for Healthy Me

From Darkness to En-Lighted

Have you ever entered an area that is pitch dark? Most of us have found ourselves in such areas at least once in our lives —areas that if there were just the smallest amount of light, we'd be able to avoid collisions and feel less lost. In these pitch-dark scenarios, we often get distracted by or duped into seeking light from others. These people may be sources of light, but they are often NOT the light that is appropriate or meant for our unique needs.

One of our main challenges during such times is to recognize that the most sound and accurate light is within us. In fact, for every myth and every odyssey written, the (s)hero comes to realize that the answer to all riddles and the source of their strength to overcome challenges exists within him/herself. All who seek find THIS truth; it's just a matter of time.

As we embark upon our Healthy Me voyage, it's important to realize that we carry three primary light sources: the Lighthouse, Searchlight, and Spotlight. Each light plays a distinct role in shaping who we are as individuals and how we show up in our SHIPS.

"Darkness cannot drive out darkness; only light can do that."

~ Rev. Martin Luther King, Jr.

Why is light so important? This famous quote speaks to the power of light to eliminate the problems of society. The same is true for the challenges in our lives. Light gives us the opportunity to see clearly. Even the smallest amount of light can help us begin to understand where obstacles are located and how we might start to remove them.

Darkness may have served a purpose in our past: it can act as a shield from unbearable pain. However, it's important to use our light to navigate the trauma/challenging experience so we can heal from the inside out. It's okay to use a dim spotlight to start. It's okay to move slowly in these dark and difficult spaces.

For clarity, let's examine each light source and how it contributes to our development.

Lighthouse

Our lighthouse serves as our moral compass. It helps us avoid dangerous rocks that could cause our ship to run aground or wreck. It guides us toward healthy choices.

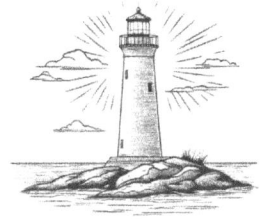

It brings us consistency and reliability. Our family and community often serve as our original lighthouses, as both help us form values. Our family keeps us safe from harm and teaches us how to navigate choppy waters. Our community shapes our cultural identity via societal norms and expectations.

Searchlight

This light serves us during periods of transition, such as when we move from relying solely on our family and community (and how others see us or expect us to be), and begin to establish who we are (our Authentic Selves).

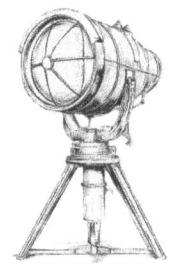

It allows us to search for our purpose and to find the meaning in our individual existence. It's a powerful light source on a swivel, which provides the flexibility necessary for making changes in our lives due to interactions with others. Our searchlight is often impacted by our need to fit in and to thrive as members of peer groups that might ultimately become our primary influence.

Actual searchlights have two major components: a lamp and a reflector. In people, the lamp represents the core friendship group with which we tend to align for support and safety. Our reflector is a mirror, and it projects our lamplight so our values, priorities, and choices can be perceived by those outside of our peer group. As we increase our watts (how brightly we shine) and creativity (how we use our light), we learn, and our searchlight changes.

Spotlight

This condensed beam of light illuminates a single spot. It's what makes us visible to the world. When a spotlight is used on a stage, it illuminates a specific area or person.

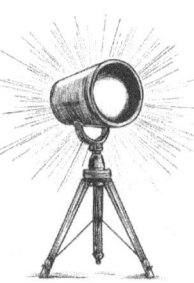

Likewise, we can use it to spotlight ourselves or our past. Because our spotlights are customized for us, they will likely give a warped or skewed perspective on others. So, one important rule about spotlights is that we don't use our spotlight to learn about other people. How might you use your lights?

Anchors - *Takeaways*

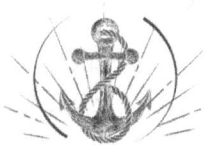

- When we're in the dark, we often seek light wherever we find it, even if the source isn't appropriate or meant for our unique needs.
- Our lighthouse serves as our moral compass and drives our decisions and priorities.
- Our searchlight is lit by our need to "fit in" and thrive as members of peer groups.
- Our personal spotlight is custom-built for our use. We can't use it on anyone else.

Your Brain in Love: Inseparable Co-Travelers
"Love & Hate"

Couples often blame one another for the problems they encounter in their relationship. Would that change if we understood the structure and function of the brain? Would that knowledge help us to stop blaming and start seeking to understand OURSELVES and our own contribution to the problems we encounter?

Neuroscientists study the structure and function of the brain. They've found a clear connection between gender and behavior, some of which may contribute to frustrations in relationships. Here are some of their findings:

- Women's prefrontal cortices are larger than men's. The larger prefrontal cortex gives women the capacity to make more thoughtful and planned decisions.
- Men tend to have a larger amygdala than women. The larger amygdala creates more aggressive and impulsive behaviors.
- Women have a larger hippocampus (the center of emotion, memory, and the autonomic nervous system), which allows them to remember more details about an event and to retain information for a long time.
- A smaller hippocampus in men could account for their tendency to use fewer words to express feelings to describe an event.
- Men predominantly use the right side of the brain when perceiving, leading to a big-picture perspective.
- Women predominantly use left-brain processing for information, leading to a detail-oriented perspective.
- Men's larger hypothalamus compels them to be more interested in sex than women.

These neuroscientific nuances are likely overlooked in intimate partnerships, which can lead to conflict when one partner expects the other to view the world the exact same way. That unmet expectation—that partners will agree on everything—serves as a set-up for intimate partner conflict.

In the early 1970s, there was a chart-topping song by the Persuaders entitled "A Thin Line Between Love and Hate." Most people related to the song due to its description of the emotions surrounding a break-up. The song also supports neuroscientific notions that both emotions—love and hate—are generated from the same part of the brain. This fact may lend some credence to the adage, "You can't hate someone you never loved." Although that theory has yet to be proven, what is certain is that these opposing emotions share the same pathways in the brain. Research has also shown that the area of our brain that regulates judgment and reasoning doesn't fully function whenever we experience love and hate. Think about that: whether you're in love, or whether you despise, your ability to reason and judge is impaired.

To avoid letting your emotions "drive while impaired," here are a few nuggets to consider:

- Neuroscience explains some of your partner's behavior.
- Accept that your partner does NOT see the world from your lenses. The most proactive and practical behavior for you is to manage your expectations.
- Avoid making major decisions during times of intense emotion. Rather, give yourself time/space to consider the potential impacts of your decision; stepping back will help you to maximize sound decision-making.

Start today—right now. Think of something that has you feeling extremely positively or negatively toward someone. Ask yourself: What expectations do I have about this situation?

> **Anchors** - *Takeaways*
>
>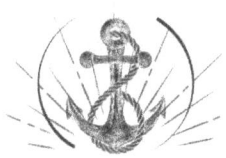
> - Trying to find partners exactly like us is futile.
> - Since we are all different, it will take effort to understand others and to be understood by others.
> - Embrace our differences and support our uniqueness.

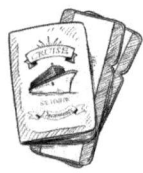

Alone, Not Lonely

For some people being alone is a reward or achievement. Consider Dan, a full-time college student and athlete. All through high school, Dan was socially well connected and considered a reliable teammate on the sports teams he joined. He was tall and handsome but never arrogant. He dated casually but never seriously with anyone.

But Dan lived for his time alone. His family had a cottage on the lake in the mountains, which was Dan's sanctuary. Whenever his busy schedule allowed it, he was off to the cottage alone. He loved to work with his own thoughts, commune with nature, and relax. He felt certain that his alone time helped him deal with the rest of his busy life.

When Dan got to college, he met Ann. She was in his philosophy class and very bright. Ann was what Dan called a social butterfly. She connected with everyone, knew everyone, and seemed happiest when she was surrounded by friends. She also had several brothers and sisters and was equally happy surrounded by her family.

Dan asked Ann out on a date, and she quickly accepted. The date was very successful. Dan was a good listener and Ann loved to talk. He found her energy interesting and totally captivating.

After several dates, Dan invited Ann to join him for an extended weekend at the cottage.

He was so excited to be able to share his special place with Ann. When they arrived at the cottage, Ann was overwhelmed with the sheer beauty of the mountains and lake. But after two days, Ann asked Dan if she could invite her siblings and a few friends to join them. He was surprised at her request and asked her why. At first, she cited how beautiful the place was and her desire to share it with her social circle. After a bit more dialog she finally announced that she was feeling lonely, even though she said Dan was great company.

Dan was shocked. He had never felt that way. He realized that his desire for alone time was something he needed but that it clearly did not serve Ann.

After Dan and Ann sat together and talked through their differences, they agreed that if their relationship was to continue, they would need to keep their communication ongoing, open, and honest. Dan was more attracted to Ann than ever and Ann appeared to be equally attracted to him, as a potential partner who could listen and demonstrate respect for their differences.

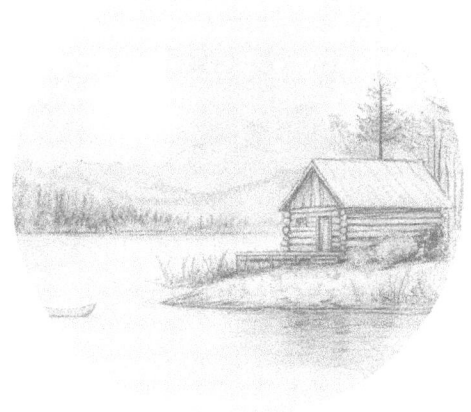

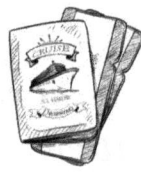

Alone But Not Lonely Continuum

As you continue your voyage toward your Authentic Self, consider the continuum below.

Like most continuum measurements, there is no good or bad. The idea is to help you realize where you plot yourself. If the placement pleases you, then you know that you can use it as a valuable perspective as you move forward. If your placement is not what you'd hoped for, then you have a clear target to begin your work.

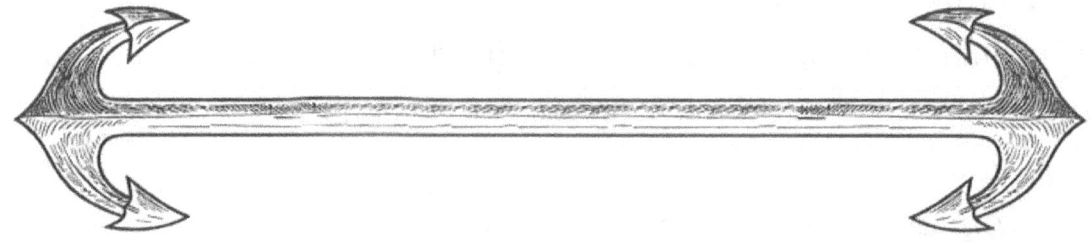

Need others around me. *Seek Solitude*
Uncomfortable when alone. *Comfortable when alone.*

INSTRUCTIONS: Place an **X** or your initials where you fall on the spectrum above. Try to think about it as *"most often"* vs. *"all the time."*

Regardless of where you placed your **X**, that position has a set of assets and a set of liabilities.

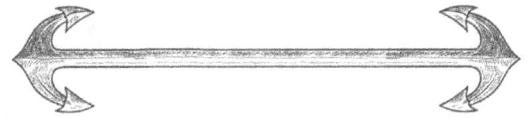

*Need others around me.
Uncomfortable when alone.*

*Seek Solitude
Comfortable when alone.*

Assets: *What are the positive outcomes from your position on the spectrum?*

_____

_____

_____

_____

_____

Liabilities: What are the unintended negative outcomes of your position?

_____

_____

_____

_____

_____

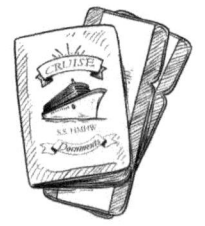 **What's My SCQ?** *(pronounced "Skew")*

What's your solitude comfort quotient (SCQ)

A key indicator of Healthy Me is your degree of comfort with your Authentic Self. This means being at ease when others aren't available to distract us from our inner thoughts, our preferred pursuits, or their expectations. This brief activity is designed to provide an idea of the degree to which you can distinguish between being ALONE and being LONELY, based on your perspective regarding solitude. Alone and lonely are two entirely different states-of-being that are often confused.

Whether it's our physical weight or the wait time for answering a phone call, it's always easier to manage what we can MEASURE. With that in mind, use the following tool to help yourself gauge what might be a recurring personal challenge: separating your <u>situation</u> from your <u>emotions</u> so you can better address BOTH.

Throughout our lives, we experience countless pressures. Many of us yield to these expectations—so much so that it becomes difficult to know and understand what we, ourselves, think and feel. One of the ways we lose sight of our authentic truth is around our emotions. Many find it difficult to distinguish and determine how we feel versus how we would describe our present situation. These two can become blurred and challenging to separate, not to mention manage.

One of the most important distinctions each of us can learn to make is the difference between being alone and being lonely. The completed survey can provide insights that help you begin making that distinction, as well as adjustments that will enable a healthier, more productive perspective on solitude and loneliness.

To determine your results, tally each column. The following page provides an explanation and insights for your tallied results.

INSTRUCTIONS: Using the options on the next page, complete the sentence, "Thinking about or being alone typically leads me to feel/behave like this..." Select one option, from either the left or right column, whichever is the most accurate for YOU most of the time.

NOTE: Once you complete this simple tool and read the descriptions of **HIGH SCQ (SCQH)**, **MODERATE SCQ (SCQM)**, and **LOW SCQ (SCQL)**, you'll see suggestions for expanding AND/OR sustaining a healthy perspective about SOLITUDE and the opportunities embedded within.

THINKING ABOUT, OR BEING, ALONE TYPICALLY LEADS ME TO FEEL/BEHAVE LIKE THIS...

FEELINGS/BEHAVIORS	FEELINGS/BEHAVIORS
Discontent	Content
Blame Self/ Others for being alone	Mental/ Physical Freedom
Feel Abandoned and or disconnected	Feel Sense of Peace
Negative Self Talk	Positive Self-Talk
Long for Proximity to Others	Leverage Solitude to Pursue Interests
Avoid Solitude	Seek Alone-Time
Going Solo or Stag = Anxiety	Going Solo or Stag = Fine
Fear Singular Activities	Welcome Singular Activities
Distract Self from Feelings when Alone	Follow My Curiosity when Alone
Need others around for Fulfillment	Find Fulfillment without Others Around

WHAT INSIGHTS DO MY RESULTS PROVIDE?
Left Column has 6 or more circled = Low SCQ = SCQL

Having a low solitude comfort quotient is NOT FATAL! Rather, it means you have tremendous opportunity to explore and develop more wholesome and positive attitudes about the VALUE of time alone. Many of us have been hoodwinked by a society that bombards us with negative images and messages regarding singular activities or time spent alone. When you read through the items in the left-hand column as a collective, they can sound as though being in the company of SELF is a bad thing!

If you scored SCQL, here's something to try the very next time you're dreading alone time:

Make a To Do list of the things you personally find fun, but you know others don't enjoy. Using your list, schedule a few of your fun items into your calendar; intentionally scheduling them for the upcoming alone-time you are presently dreading. When that alone time has passed (and you've completed your personal fun activity), make note of how you feel. Here's a sampling of positive emotions that may replace some of those negative ones you once had:

- Sense of accomplishment
- Relief due to the opportunity to focus solely on what YOU want with no others to consider
- Excited to schedule more me-time

WHAT INSIGHTS DO MY RESULTS PROVIDE?
Right Column has 6 or more circled = High SCQ = SCQH

Having a high solitude comfort quotient is a GREAT STARTING POINT! It means you likely view alone time as an opportunity packed with possibility. Where some may feel anxious if, while waiting at a restaurant, their dinner companion texts to say they are now unavailable, you might shrug off your disappointment, place your order, and start planning ways to use your time after dinner!

If you scored SCQH, here are some suggestions for maintaining your healthy perspective and feelings regarding solitude:

- Review the items that you selected from the right-side column. For each of the items selected, generate a list of REASONS those feelings/behaviors occur for you (e.g., Going solo is fine with me because I get to talk to/meet new people and that's something I really enjoy).
- Using your mobile device or desktop computer, launch your internet browser and find a free WORD CLOUD generator.
- Once you find the word cloud generator, use it to input all the statements/REASONS you generated. When you finish inputting the statements, generate the word cloud.
- Look at the word cloud generated by your entries. You'll likely see that yours is a very positive atmosphere or cloud! In fact, you may notice that the word cloud reflects how solitude is helping to FEED YOUR SOUL... and who can't do with a bit of soul food?! (See sample word cloud below). Keep it up!

WHAT INSIGHTS DO MY RESULTS PROVIDE?
Columns have equal number of items circled = Moderate SCQ = SCQM

Having a moderate solitude comfort quotient is TYPICAL. Most of us welcome solitude sometimes and find it somewhat unsettling at others (THINK: first time alone in a new home). Experiencing feelings of joy or anxiety when alone may, for you, be situational and not necessarily as predictable as it might be for those with SCQL or SCQH.

Because your SCQ may lean either high or low depending on the situation, you should seek to better understand your comfort and discomfort. For instance, being perfectly comfortable ignoring your guests at a surprise party thrown on your behalf might represent being too comfortable making others uncomfortable! Similarly, feeling so stressed and anxious that you wait inside your car for your dinner companion might signal more SCQL than your balanced results indicate. Only YOU can judge, and it requires honest exploration of the reasons you are comfortable or anxious.

If you've managed to maintain a relatively balanced perspective about solitude and the positive impact it can yield, try reducing some of the stressors that might creep in those times you are facing solitude by implementing suggestions from the SCQL and/or SCQH profile recommendations.

Whatever you do, avoid being too hard on yourself. Society bombards us with negative messages regarding singular activities or time spent alone.

Knowing why we feel what we feel is the antidote to behaving according to societal expectations. Here are some questions to ask yourself so you can further explore and achieve even more clarity about your WHYs:

- Do I tag along with others because I enjoy being with them, or because I would rather do the activity with others, even if I don't like them? Why?
- When I have errands or chores, do I intentionally invite another/others to join me for the company? Why?
- Is it difficult for me to spend an entire weekend alone? Why?
- Can I experience happiness when I am alone? Why?
- Will I try new things alone if there is no one to join me? Why?

What Does it All Mean?

There is no right or wrong or good or bad associated with where you placed your X on the continuum. There is a great deal of value in knowing your score and how you decide to manage it. Once it becomes clear for you, it is another valuable guide as you plot your voyage forward.

Anchors - *Takeaways*

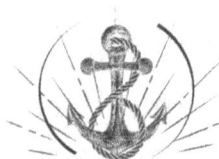

- Your SCQ provides valuable insight into your past and current relationships.
- Knowing the difference between being alone and being lonely helps us manage our expectations of ourselves and others.
- Once we understand that there is a difference between alone and lonely, we are better positioned to communicate more clearly with others.

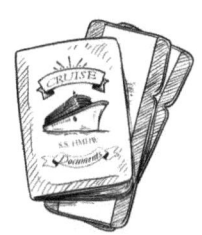

Barnacles and Rust or Why Do Some of My Relationships End Badly?

Where Do Our Barnacles Come From (and where do we hide them)?

We all have barnacles. Like the ones that attach themselves to the underside of boats, our barnacles are everywhere and can attach without you even knowing about it—or being able to see them until you look beneath the surface. We can define barnacles as life lessons, beliefs, or ideas that you have accumulated over time that may not serve you any longer. They feel like a part of you, but they are merely attached to you. Like the live aquatic version, if we don't care for and remove our barnacles, they slow down our journey and can even alter our ability to steer.

Searching for barnacles isn't easy. It requires courage and objective introspection, or the ability to look honestly within. But the payoff is worth the discomfort as you continue the journey to your Authentic Self. Let's look at some of the more obvious places where barnacles can and will attach.

Family:

Sometimes the lessons taught to us by our families, while well intentioned, can slow us down as adults. In many ways, adolescence is a developmental period wherein we examine the lessons we've learned so far. Ideas of gender identity, religion, race, and even intelligence can all slow us down as we try to sort out what we've been taught versus who we really are.

Practical Examples:

- Caregivers/family members who warn children against friending seemingly disruptive peers.
- Encouragement to eat everything on your plate.
- Parents cannot, or should not, be disobeyed.
- Our family does things the right way.

Standard Education:

Good, professional teachers maintain strong control over their classrooms with positive intent. Many well-managed classrooms have lots of rules. Some of those rules remain with us as we move through our educational journey. We should examine them to see if they help us or slow us down.

Practical Examples:

- Always work independently.
- Memorize dates and names.
- The teacher must never be challenged.

Our Social Circle:

Since it is important to most of us to be a part of a social circle of friends and confidants, we need to accept some barnacles to stay a member of the group. Examining the spoken and unspoken rules of a group can often lead to the discovery that membership has slowed down our journey. The group seeks to hold its place in society while you seek to continue to grow.

Practical Examples:

- Our group should be exclusively White, Black, Republican, Democrat, etc.
- Showing allegiance to the group is more important than understanding the values the group holds.
- The members of our group deserve special attention.

Social Media:

Unfortunately, virtually anything can appear on social media without regard for accuracy. There is minimal fact-checking. Opinion is expressed as fact, and facts are presented as opinion.

Practical Examples:

- World leaders, celebrities, etc., have been falsely reported dead multiple times.
- The people who attacked the Capitol on January 6, 2021 viewed themselves as patriots.
- Trends in behavior, attire, and musical tastes are provided by "influencers" with little or no validation that they are popular.

Our Past Relationships:

Perhaps one of the easier places for barnacles to grow is within our past relationships, especially if that relationship ended due to a conflict. The things that our partners found difficult to deal with tend to feel permanent.

Practical Examples:

- "The differences in our religion (or politics, fashion, education, etc.) mean that we can't remain together."
- "I expect you to put me ahead of your family or past relationships."
- "We've grown too far apart to repair the damage."

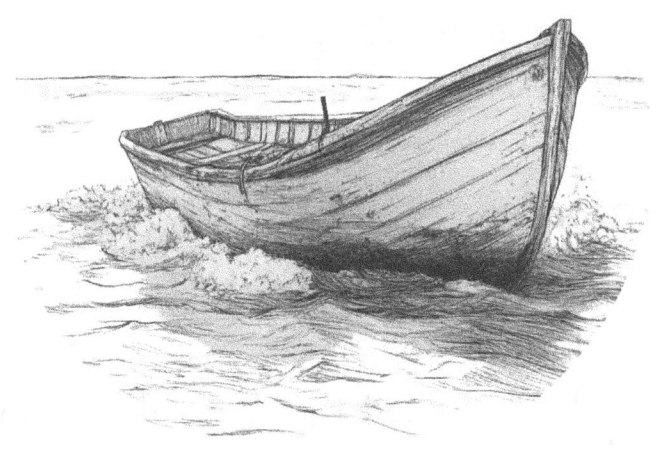

From Barnacles to Rust

We've had a chance to explore the idea of barnacles as experiences, events, and beliefs in our life that ultimately slow down our journey—and while difficult, these barnacles are much easier to manage than rust.

Rust is much more destructive than barnacles. Barnacles attach to us from the outside, but rust hurts us from within. Getting rid of rust is a much more elaborate process. Trying to ignore rust is dangerous because rust spreads unless it is treated. Here's an example:

> *We know of a woman who experienced a wonderful childhood, filled with love and growth. She was taught to accept all people, regardless of differences. Central to that supportive childhood was her relationship with her father. She idolized her dad and he felt the same way toward her.*
>
> *While visiting home from college, the woman thought it would be a nice surprise for her father if she cleaned and organized his bedroom closet. What she found threw her into a spin of uncertainty and despair.*
>
> *For there, hanging in the farthest back corner of his closet, were her father's Ku Klux Klan robes. The markings on the robes indicated that her dad was a leader of his chapter.*

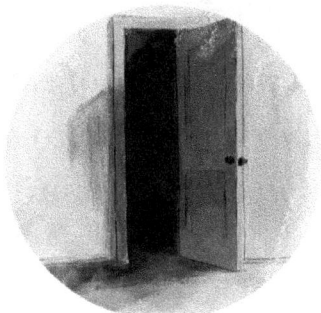

That's the kind of power that rust has in our quest for a Healthy Me and our Authentic Self. In that story, our friend knew she had a lot of work to do, decisions to make, painful areas to explore, and relationships to change or potentially lose altogether. Maybe her first thought was to try to ignore what she found, but soon she realized that she could not be true to herself if she left this situation unresolved.

Once we are aware of rust in our lives, we cannot continue onward as we were before we knew about the rust. Our ship must go into dry dock for repair. Without that, we risk sinking.

Facing those areas of rust, of situations and information so powerful that they can stop our journey, is at best a risky business. In his book The Five Questions, author Dr. John Scherer offers this illustrative example of what that risk looks like:

> *You are walking alone on a jungle path. Suddenly you look up and see a tiger coming toward you. What do you do? Of course, for most of us the first reaction is "Run, Run, Run". But let's view things from the tiger's eyes... When the tiger sees you, he isn't certain what you are when you are facing him; but if you turn and run, then he sees you as... LUNCH! No doubt he will chase and catch you.*
>
> *Facing him isn't any guarantee of safety, either. Yet the outcome is less certain compared to running away from the tiger. If any safe solution exists, it'll come from facing the tiger.*

That's the way rust works as we travel toward our Authentic Self. Running from or trying to ignore the rusty situation will not work. In many cases it'll make the situation worse. Consider the example of our friend and her father's KKK robes. If she tries to ignore it, surely her relationship with her dad will suffer, and he'll recognize the change without knowing why. While there are no guarantees that they will resolve this situation successfully, their odds are much better if they try.

Steps to Managing Rust:

- Identify the situation, event, or condition that is stopping your journey. Look at it as thoroughly and objectively as you can.
- Identify what is at stake if you address this rust.
- Decide on a course of action. Generally it's best to try and resolve the issue. Do not blame, shame, or try to guilt the other person(s). Your goal is identifying the rust, removing it, and resuming your journey to your best Authentic Self.

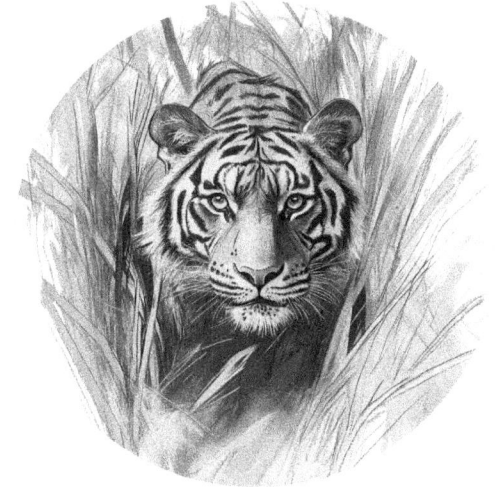

Anchors - *Takeaways*

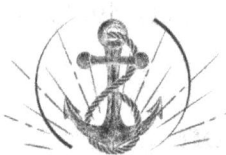

- As we journey through life, we collect barnacles that have the potential to limit our progress toward Authentic Self/Healthy Me.
- If we don't tend to our barnacles and rust, we can lose the ability to steer or change course.
- The most effective/healthy practice is to objectively identify and address whatever is sticking to you so that your journey for Authentic Self isn't weighed down with extra baggage or blown off course.
- The solution to managing your barnacles is inside you, there is NO OTHER WAY TO MANAGE THEM.

"None of us can change the past, but all of us can LEARN from it."

~ C. Grayson, 2023

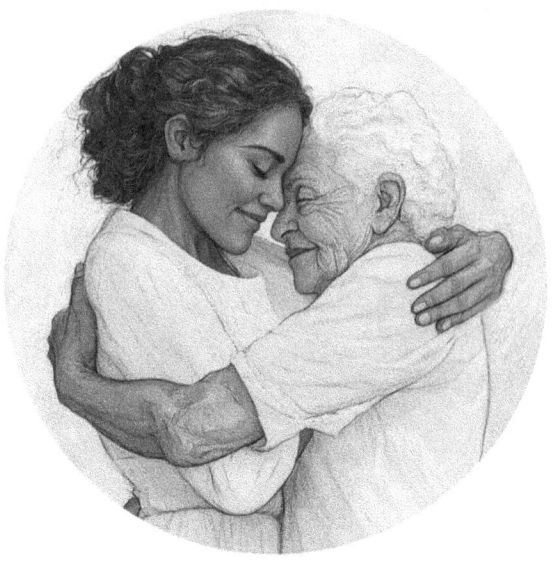

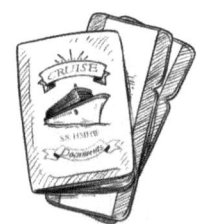

A.W.O.L. – 3 Ship Rules to Help YOU Stop Running

AWOL is a military term that stands for Absent Without Official Leave. Among non-military folks, AWOL has come to signify someone who goes away without taking the proper or established steps to do so. In other words, it's essentially "ghosting." In relationships, this describes someone who avoids or abandons problems and leaves other(s) hanging.

Some of us have been AWOL from our Authentic Self. If you are, you may go through your days not realizing you're wearing a mask: the mask of the persona you want the world to see but is NOT who you really are.

These folks have not learned to address their challenges; they create substitutes like shopping or chasing new relationships to feel better because constant masquerading is draining! We fill our lives with trivial pursuits to avoid the most important pursuit of all: finding our Authentic Self. Unfortunately, these substitutes never bring the satisfaction that comes from knowing and loving that Self. We eventually tire of toys or other pursuits and are left with emptiness heaped atop everything from which we were running: our own draining inauthenticity.

SHIP RULE No.1
*No matter how far we move from our last partner,
or how frequently we change hairstyles and wardrobes,
we cannot run from our own baggage.*

Relationships don't fix people, nor do they help us forget about our last heartbreak. On the contrary, intimate partnerships expose both our strengths and vulnerabilities. They tend to accelerate the collision between our baggage and reality. Because happiness is an inside job, no one can make us happy but us. On the other hand, relationships provide an opportunity to share our happiness with others we deem special. Relationships help us connect with others and, if possible, share ourselves.

SHIP RULE No.2
Things and other people don't complete us or make us whole.

No matter how much our parents may have sheltered us, or how careful we've been as adults, we all carry leftover pieces of the past. Our goal is to not run away from that baggage but instead to unpack it piece by piece, examine it, and decide whether to salvage it or let it go. This approach is the gateway for bringing our healthiest and best self to our relationships. Our first action, therefore, is to stop running.

Stop

To continuously work toward Healthy Me and to practice Healthy We , you must let go of your defenses and excuses. Look in the mirror and identify what you must start unpacking. If you have a partner, don't concern yourself with whether they, too, are unpacking—what's in their bag is their personal work. When, if ever, they begin unpacking is their decision.

Reflect

Once you start unpacking and examining your baggage, you may recognize a repeating pattern in your relationships. If the pattern is a negative one, ask yourself what you need to do to break the pattern, change the trajectory, and improve the outcomes.

Respond

To optimize your results, complete this book in the sequence it was written. Avoid skipping around because you might overlook key areas of the process by assuming that a section doesn't apply to you. Take it all in, as intended, so you can address root causes with long-term solutions rather than short-term patch-ups. Stop looking for quick fixes—you're not broken. You just require your undivided attention.

SHIP RULE No.3
*No matter how fast or how far we run,
none of us can outrun OURSELVES.*

How to stop running

Get started by honestly answering these questions:

- What do I tend to avoid in my relationships?
- What am I running from in my life?
- What are the themes in my relationships?

To maintain momentum, remember:

It's time to stop blaming others for your unhappiness. Start unpacking your stuff to let healing begin. Over time, hard work lightens your bags!

Anchors - *Takeaways*

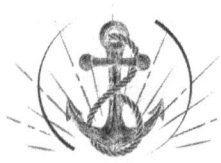

- Stop running from yourself.
- Stop blaming others for patterns of unhappiness in your life.
- Start unpacking YOUR stuff.

DECK 1

EXPLORE DECK

Explore Deck

EXPLORE is the first component of the Healthy Me process. When we explore, we uncover all the secrets that have been buried and acknowledge the hurt that has existed in our life. You're not having a pity party but are instead facing the music; you're working through the trauma that you've been exposed to without blaming, shaming, or excusing your situation. Exploration and excavation start with asking ourselves: What's keeping us from healthy?

To explore, suggests that we remove the bandages from our wounds and start the healing process rather than allow the sores to further fester.

Exploration is important because the more aware we are aware of our trauma, bruises, and scars, the more work we can do to discover our Authentic Self.

When you're ready, dive deeper:
Get started by honestly answering these questions:
- What are the recurring themes in my life?
- What am I running from?
- Which areas do I need to enhance or improve?

In terms of the bigger picture, how does Healthy Me contribute to Healthy We ? When most couples get together, they bring individual baggage and far too little insight about how their partner's behaviors and choices may trigger their own past trauma and unresolved issues. The conflict cycle is typically perpetual with no resolution, causing each partner to build a wall of defense from further hurt.

This triggers each to look for the problem outside of themselves rather than looking within. What's more, most couples are unequipped to effectively deal with conflict because they are out of touch with their baggage. Exploring takes self-discipline and self-awareness. We must be willing to be vulnerable to explore. We must be willing to hear things that we may not want to hear to gain insight about the barriers that keep us from reaching and living as our Authentic Self. We must also be willing to be still when we don't know what to do. This means we must avoid fleeing from our hurts and isolating ourselves from others.

We must stand tall outside of our comfort zones to get the answers we need to move forward. We must identify how we've concealed our past hurts so that we can address and heal them now. We must speak our truth in OUR OWN VOICE.

To dive deeper, ask:

- What behaviors do I engage in to distract me from my trauma and hurt?
- Are these behaviors healthy and moving me towards my Authentic Self or are these behaviors destructive and separating me further from my truth?
- How do I spend my time?
- What's important to ME?

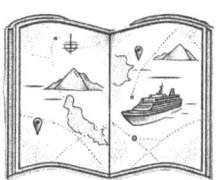

Charter - *Getting REAL: The Value of Vulnerability*

(Ready, Set, Let's Be Vulnerable)

Many of us value resiliency. We strive to demonstrate it and, rightfully, reward it in others. Yet we often consider resiliency to be a stand-alone aspect of a person and fail to acknowledge that resiliency has a behavioral cousin called vulnerability: the act of exposing oneself to hurt, rejection, and other forms of physical or emotional hazards. While none of us seeks to be harmed, being vulnerable is critical for relationships. It is the very strongest who willingly share their vulnerabilities to establish and maintain healthy bonds with others.

For example, back in the 1990s, Real Life was a reality TV show that featured young adults who were learning about life while sharing a house and navigating relationships. During their collective journey, each was forced to face their own baggage. As the season unfolded, most of the cast learned the value of being real with each other versus hiding behind an imaginary mask of what others expected.

Valuable life lessons from the show were:

- Being vulnerable with others can be scary, but it's necessary for personal and interpersonal growth.
- Before we can be real with others, we must own our experiences without romanticizing them because only FICTIONAL CHARACTERS have happily-ever-after endings.
- Some of us have been through a lot, and we have the physical and/or emotional scars to show it.
- Being real doesn't mean we seek to demonstrate how tough we are but rather that we learned from our experiences and embrace the Authentic Self we discovered due to those experiences.

One common question about being vulnerable is, "How can I get started when what I'm masking is painful, embarrassing, and/or may disappoint others?" Here are a few ways.

Non-apologetic acceptance of YOUR OWN STORY.

Own it. Start by practicing acceptance; your past does not define you. Understanding our beginnings allows us to accurately measure our progress. Imagine that your life began with a starting point, like a race with hurdles. It would be impossible to know how far you've traveled if, despite days of travel, your starting line remained beneath your feet. Flaws, missteps, setbacks, and occasionally getting blown off course are common experiences. Also realize that being real and vulnerable won't erase the past but it allows us to let go of guilt, shame, and self-blame. Emotional vulnerability also demonstrates inner strength: willingness to risk sharing yourself with others despite having no control over their reaction/response regarding your authenticity.

The British mystery novelist Daniel Hurst says, "If the plan doesn't work, change the plan, but never the GOAL." It's a great concept and terrific advice because vulnerable, real people stay true to their goals and adjust, as they learn and find it necessary, to get closer to the finish line. Do you know what you want? Do you know where you're going? Are you working towards something bigger than you? Real people are not chameleons; we don't change who we are to adapt to others' expectations.

Be open to what you learn about yourself. Never fear looking into the mirror and studying your reflection. As you embrace your Authentic Self, you'll likely detect alignment in various areas of your life: spiritual, intellectual, emotional, social, and even financial alignment. Examination of your reflection may reveal a key that's been long missing and can unlock a door of possibilities.

Squash the negative self-talk. It sabotages your future by drawing negative people to you. While others may not understand your realness, don't allow their lack of understanding or support to thwart you! Being connected to others and sharing your best You requires imaginary ear plugs to block out naysaying, skepticism, and undermining—especially your own. Emotional vulnerability means you are strong enough to share your truths and withstand the doubt others express.

> *""Vulnerability is the birthplace of love, belonging, joy, courage, empathy, and creativity."*
> *~ Brene Brown"*

Remember, society impacts all of us even though the impact may manifest differently. Many men find difficulty in being vulnerable with their intimate partners and families due to social gender expectations. Despite the inherent strength and wisdom of acknowledging fears/concerns, conventional society conflates vulnerability with weakness when the practice is exhibited by men. Knowing this should position us to encourage men's expression of vulnerability and wholeheartedly support it. For example, because some people may find it more challenging to let others know what's really going on in their lives (be it financial, career, or health related), a key indication of a healthy couple is that they create a space for each other to fearlessly share their vulnerabilities without being shamed or embarrassed.

Are you 4 R.E.A.L.?

R – Raw (Natural state vs Processed/Masked)
E – Expressive (Willing to communicate)
A – And
L – Liberated (Free from others' expectations)

Notice that our acronym R.E.A.L. matches the intentional alternate spelling of REALationships in the book title. We are deliberately reinforcing the concept that healthy relationships are characterized by their REAL-ness. So the next time you read healthy relationship, feel free to substitute REALationship—and know that you're describing a dynamic that is truthful, open, and unfettered by society's assumptions!

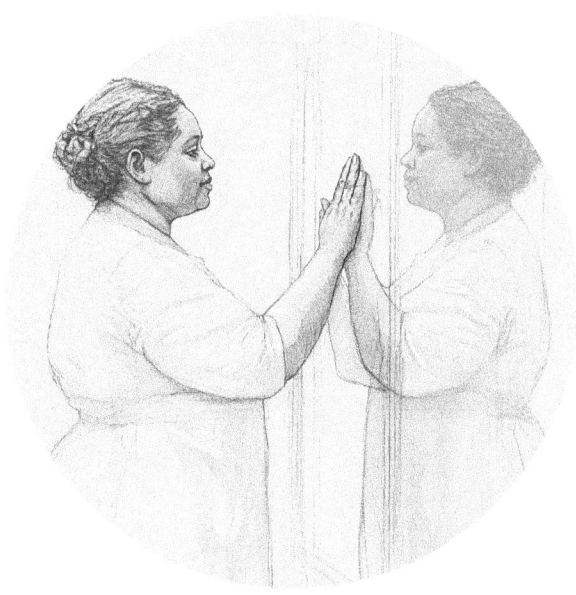

Anchors - *Takeaways*

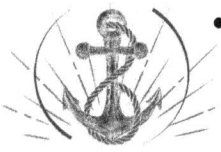

- Resiliency has a behavioral cousin called vulnerability: the act of exposing oneself to hurt, rejection, and other forms of physical or emotional hazards.
- Your past does not define you. Understanding our beginning allows us to accurately measure our progress.
- Vulnerable, real people (versus fictional characters) stay true to their goals and adjust, as they learn and find it necessary, to get closer to the finish line.
- Never fear looking into the mirror and studying your reflection.
- While others may not understand your realness, don't allow their lack of understanding and support to thwart you.

Excursion 1 - Reflect on My Vulnerability

1. Identify the people in your life with whom you can be emotionally vulnerable.

_____
_____
_____
_____
_____

2. What have you been holding onto in fear of being misunderstood or rejected?

_____
_____
_____
_____
_____

Excursion 1 cont.- Reflect on My Vulnerability

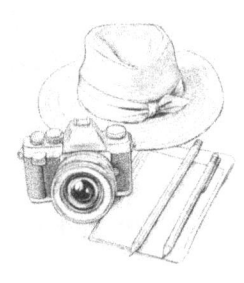

3. What steps do you plan to take to become more emotionally vulnerable with others?

_____
_____
_____
_____
_____

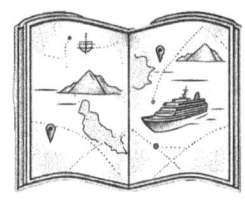

Charter - *Ongoing Journey to Find & Understand Your Authentic Me*

"Owning our [personal] story can be hard but not nearly as difficult as spending our lives running from it. [...]Only when we are brave enough to explore the darkness will we discover the infinite power of our light."

~Brené Brown

Everything we do boils down to this: stimulus and response. Each response brings us closer to, or takes us further from, our goal. On this voyage to discover our Authentic Self, we'll start unpacking whatever it is we're carrying.

The Brené Brown quote regarding courageously exploring, owning, and addressing those aspects of our individual stories upon which we build our lives is both insightful AND prescriptive. We are going to get started by unpacking your baggage. You'll learn ways to accept and heal issues that may be obstructing your full potential. As you accept and heal, you're better prepared to grow. All of this provides what you need to understand, accept, and present who you are—your *Authentic Self*.

When you commit to addressing your baggage, you commit to looking at difficult subjects. It's critical to examine the impact of the past and acknowledge the connection between past trauma/events. For instance, how that trauma and or those events are triggered in our daily life; and the traps we fall into when we ignore how the traps impact our relationships. For those who are committed to understanding themselves, looking back can provide an opportunity to see what worked/helped successfully navigate those challenging waters. Completing a T3 assessment provides you with a new perspective—a perspective that can be used to understand yourself and your unique challenges. Having the courage to lean into possible discomfort and fear when exploring is critical in becoming more and more authentic.

Your T3 assessment will help you uncover strengths and skills that have served you well in the past and that you can apply now and onward. During exploration, you may gain awareness of past traumas and their triggers; as you continue to dig deeper, you can empower yourself with healthy choices for addressing the T3 results you discover.

To start unpacking and identifying what you're bringing on your journey, it will be helpful to ask yourself questions like:

- How have my past experiences shaped me?
- What are some of my emotionally painful childhood experiences?
- Where were the moments of joy in my childhood experiences?
- Why do I do the things I do?
- What are my relationships with my children and family?
- How might I characterize past intimate partnerships?
- What's keeping me from achieving Healthy Me?
- What components of Healthy Me do I already have?
- Which recurring themes in my life continue to surface again and again?
- What am I running from?
- What are my scabs and scars?

There are no incorrect responses to the questions above or the assessment below, because each will help you identify some of your emotional wounds or how you have healed them. It is, however, important for you to be aware of what you are feeling and to explore the origins of those feelings. You will have multiple opportunities to develop healthy strategies for working through your traumas, triggers, and traps.

The T3 assessment is the first step in identifying your unique work to achieve Healthy Me. As such, take care not to overwhelm yourself with trying to understand and "correct" your life experiences using just one charter or tool. The T3 assessment serves as both a starting point and reference: It keeps your issues focused and helps you tackle your specific work. As you engage in your work, you may identify additional traumas, triggers, and traps. That's part of the ongoing process: pursuing Healthy Me never ends because the more you discover about yourself, the more you'll seek to understand.

One final point: you can use your T3 Response Sheet as a checklist of the "stuff" you carry in your bags. Rummaging and sifting through your life-stuff is the best way to sustain Healthy Me and unapologetically embrace your Authentic Self.

Anchors - *Takeaways*

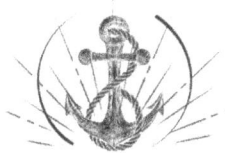

- Assessing your traumas, triggers, and traps is a first step for discovering your Authentic Self.
- Your T3 results help to chart the course or pathway to broadening your understanding of your Authentic Self and what's needed to maintain Healthy Me.

Excursion 2.   T3 Assessment

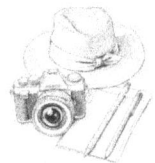

STATEMENT	AGREEMENT RATING			
TRAUMA	STRONGLY AGREE	AGREE	DISAGREE	STRONGLY DISAGREE
I have phobias or pet peeves whose origins cannot be pinpointed				
I rely on/use a chemical or herbal method to achieve a state of relaxation				
I often feel depressed and cannot pinpoint the reason(s)				
I have disturbing dreams that are recurrent				
I find that discussing certain past life events feels frightening				
I have no memory of large chunks of your life				

STATEMENT	AGREEMENT RATING			
TRIGGERS	STRONGLY AGREE	AGREE	DISAGREE	STRONGLY DISAGREE
There specific situations that result in my uncontrollable anger				
I clearly describe the type of situations that bring on feelings of vulnerability or feelings of being unsafe				
The very thought of attending certain events makes me feel uneasy				
The very thought of certain people makes me feel negative feelings				

STATEMENT	AGREEMENT RATING			
TRAPS	STRONGLY AGREE	AGREE	DISAGREE	STRONGLY DISAGREE
Despite having confronted the issues, the same arguments crop up				
Ignoring recurring issues only makes me angrier				
Trying to repress my anger about a situation makes me feel worse				
I de-escalate conflicts by walking away from the situation				
After I express my anger/disappointment, I shut down discussion of the topic				
My anger toward others is typically due to something they've done to me				

Excursion 3 - T3 Response Sheet

Instructions: Based on your T3 Assessment, complete the worksheet for those statements receiving Agreement Ratings of Strongly Agree or Agree. You can leave the rest blank.

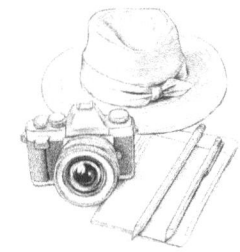

Trauma

- Identify phobias and pet peeves –

- Ways you self-medicate –

- Depression moments –

- Subject of recurrent dreams –

- Phases of life with no to minimum memory –

Triggers

- The type of situations that cause me anger –

- Ways that I feel vulnerable –

- Social events that cause negative feelings –

- People that cause negative feelings–

- External (symbols, music, places, etc.) that cause negative feelings –

Traps

- What are the reccurent conflicts? –

- What issues do you tend to ignore? –

- What issues do you tend to repress? –

- In upcoming Charters, you will more deeply explore the above assessment.

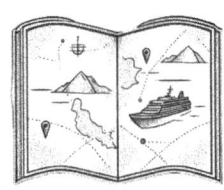 **Charter** - *Healing Points*

All of us are vulnerable to emotional wounds as we go through our life journey. These wounds are often unintentionally caused by people close to us, like our parents and other family members; intended or not these wounds can have a negative impact on us. We try to hide these wounds from others by wearing a mask that conveys we are okay. However, the reality is that many of us are silently suffering, which results in the perpetuation of unhealthy relationships. The good news is that emotional wounds can also be healing points that serve as restorative elements in our lives.

"I know this mask is uncomfortable and holding me back--time for me to take it off...

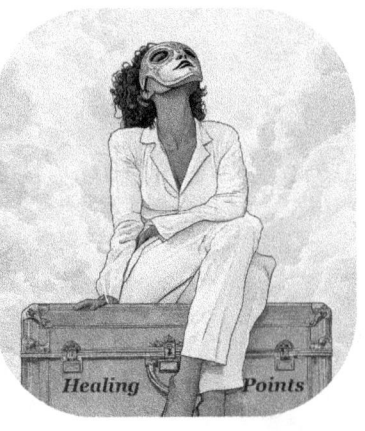

but I don't know where to put it?"

Discerning the difference between trauma triggers and healing points can be confusing because they are related but not necessarily the same. For example, we can be triggered by someone's yelling, but our healing point is knowing that this yelling brings up the feelings that we are misunderstood and voiceless.

Our healing points provide an opportunity to repair emotional wounds as we work toward Healthy Me. Healing points are connected to our overall health and should be addressed so we can establish a healthy lifestyle. The goal, however, is not to fix the past or rehash past trauma but to bring ourselves to a place of homeostasis or balance.

Remember, we all enter our relationships carrying our own baggage. Many of us don't know what's in our bag and feel more comfortable hiding it from ourselves and others. Yet to truly achieve a Healthy Me, we must take our bag out from under the bed (or wherever we've stuffed it), open it up, and begin to face those things in our life that have kept us from Healthy Me.

Know that you are not alone: we all must go through this process to get to our best ME. We all must take a bold step to transform our wounds into acknowledged healing points.

In 1998, Canadian singer Alanis Morissette released her song "Thank You" from her fourth album. The song emphasizes the importance of accepting life's challenges to move people closer to their healing. It also stresses NOT running from or deflecting our truth, but rather embracing our hardships as transformative, with an attitude of gratitude and purpose. The same is true in working towards Healthy Me.

Anchors - *Takeaways*

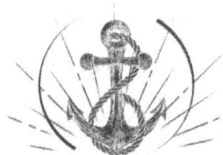

- Healing points are opportunities to repair emotional wounds.
- We ALL carry baggage, whether or not we admit it.
- The first step to healing is identifying our healing points.

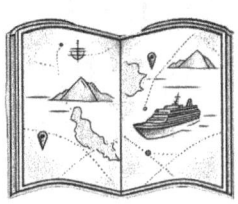

Charter -*Our Primary Color*
(Examine, Evaluate, and Ensure Alignment)

In the T3 Activity we asked you to EXPLORE yourself.

Among your early crew of influencers, some may have been more influential than others. Imagine that your early influencers were tubes of paint, squeezed onto an artist's palette. The colors that were the earliest and most abundant are YOUR PRIMARY COLORS. Depending on how we mix primary colors, we can form many other colors beyond red, blue, and yellow.

In the story below, Dave was able to take some of his dad's teachings, some of his mom's teachings, and some of his grandfather's teachings. Depending on how much of each "color" Dave mixes, he will create a color that is uniquely his own and reflects his own thoughts, feelings, and beliefs. The point: we have primary and secondary influences on our Authentic Self. Taking time to identify who and what those influences were provides insight and opportunity for better understanding of ourselves.

Here's an example of how the process might play out:

Dave was considered a good athlete even as a young boy. This was no surprise since his father was very athletic and renowned for his prowess on the playing fields. Despite his small size, Dave could hold his own in a football or baseball game with bigger boys due to his quickness and smart play—he was adept at figuring out the best way to win.

Dave was devoted to his father. His dad was his coach in all things athletic, and Dave was happy to have his guidance. When Dave got to high school and made the football team, his father told him how proud he was. At that point, Dad told Dave that if he expected to win at sports, he must view his opponent as his enemy—someone you must not just beat, but destroy.

This guidance felt wrong to Dave. His opponents were often his friends off the field, and while he clearly wanted to win when they were his opponents, he couldn't reconcile the idea of destroying them. This notion created a position hard for Dave to maintain without, seemingly, harming his relationship with his dad. Dave also felt that he couldn't share his dilemma with his mother because she would staunchly resist the "destroy your opponent" approach. This was a dilemma because it made Dave the pickle-in-the-middle between Mom and Dad.

So, Dave waited. His sports performances were solid, but he was not a superstar, despite constant encouragement from Dad. Dave eventually decided to confide in his grandfather, with whom he had a close and loving relationship.

Gramps listened carefully and asked a few clarifying questions but didn't tell Dave what to do.

Instead, he told Dave that it was time for him to find his own path. Gramps encouraged Dave to explore this and other lessons to be sure that they aligned with not only who Dave really was, but also who Dave wanted to be. "Welcome to growing up!" was Gramp's guidance.

Notice that there is neither anger nor negative confrontation in Dave's story. He instinctively recognized that the well-meaning motives which drove his influencers were designed to guide his development.

In the Excursion below, you'll take some time to explore and examine your own primary and secondary influences. What lessons did you learn? Are any of those lessons fact, opinion, relevant, and/or obsolete?

> ### **Anchors** - *Takeaways*
>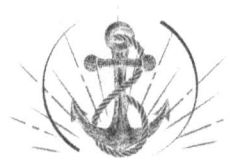
> - Well-meaning primary and secondary influencers helped us develop.
> - Some of the lessons taught to us have outlasted their relevance.
> - It is up to each of us to constantly explore and examine our lessons to determine what to preserve and what is no longer a valid fit for our Authentic Self/Healthy Me.

Excursion 4 - Questions to Guide Your Exploration & Examination
(They Key to unlock your understanding of you)

Instructions: Using the parable of Dave on the previous pages, review the process Dave used to identify and assess input from his primary and secondary influencers. Place Dave's answers to each question on the corresponding line below. After practicing with Dave's assessment, try answering the questions for yourself.

Step 1: Look at the illustration below: The primary colors represent those initial, formative influencers (red, yellow, and blue). You'll notice an overlap that creates another set of colors: the secondary colors. In this illustration, green, violet, and orange are the secondary colors.

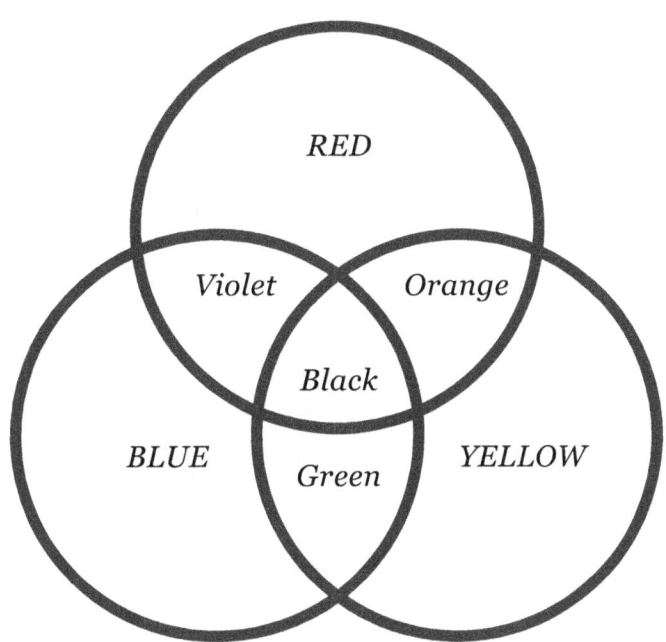

Step 2: Complete the worksheet. Practice first with Dave's story, then complete the worksheet for yourself.

Q1: What were Dave's influences from his mom?
Place in the Blue Space

_____

Q2: What were Dave's influences from his dad?
Place in the Red Space

_____

Q3: What were Dave's influences from his grandpa?
Place in the Yellow Space

_____

Q4: What influence(s) outside of Dave's family may have reinforced the influence from Grandpa and Dad?
Place in the Orange Space

_____

Q5: What influence(s) outside of Dave's family may have reinforced the influences received from Mom and Dad?
Place in the Violet Space

_____

Q6: What were Dave's influences from his grandpa and Mom?
Place in the Green Space

_____

Q7: As Dave examine(d) his comfort and leanings, what may have been his own, unique interest(s)/pathway?
Place in the Black Space

_____

Step 3: Answer the same seven questions for yourself. Because your story is different from Dave's, your primary and secondary influences will be different (e.g., not necessarily Mom/Dad/Grandpa). Think about your influences so you'll arrive at *your TRUTH*.

Q1: What were your influences from your mom or another guardian?
Place in the Blue Space

_____

_____

Q2: What were your influences from your dad or another guardian?
Place in the Red Space

_____

_____

Q3: What were your influences from your grandparents or other relatives?
Place in the Yellow Space

_____

_____

Q4: What influence(s) outside of your family may have reinforced the influence from your grandparents and father?
Place in the Orange Space

_____

_____

Q5: What influences may have reinforced the influences received from your Mom and Dad?
Place in the Violet Space

_____

_____

_____

_____

Q6 : What were the influences from your grandparents/ relatives and Mom.
Place in the Green Space

_____

_____

_____

_____

Q7: As you examine your comforts and leanings, what are your own, unique interest(s)/pathways?
Place in the Black Space

_____

_____

_____

_____

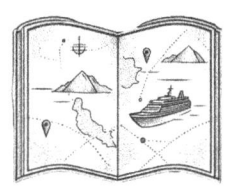 **Charter** *-Legacy, Patterns, & Generational Cycles*

Have you ever pulled out an old pair of jeans or a jacket you no longer wear and, upon reaching into a pocket, found items or cash you've long forgotten? If what you find is money, you tend to feel pretty good about it, even lucky. Finding a piece of jewelry can make you feel like you've struck gold. But what happens when you find other items—items that represent negative experiences and bad memories? What if you pull out tissues used during a funeral, or the phone number of a former friend? Do you feel as fortunate with these finds?

Looking back on the events that have impacted your life is like reaching into those old jeans: you're bound to find some good and bad things. You may have totally forgotten the details of events, but their impact on you is their LEGACY. Your mind is a treasure trove of information that can be accessed and converted to knowledge; this knowledge can be the basis of your WISDOM about YOU. Unfortunately, most people want to dispose of the bad while glorifying the good.

Everything you find can be used for good IF you're willing to honestly examine it and objectively ask: How did this impact the ME I am today? Don't suppress what you find. If your answers sound like: pretending that it never happened, refusing to come to terms with the issue(s), or burying the memory(ies), you may want to pause and look deeper. Repressing often leads to us stumbling over these memories again when we encounter similar experiences or feelings (aka being triggered). This recall is often unconscious and can compel us to behave in ways that even we, ourselves, neither understand nor recognize.

IF we are willing to be courageous and dig into our past, we can unearth hidden secrets and hurts. We can empower ourselves to face those life events that keep our Authentic Self in hiding. We can put down our mask and FREE OURSELVES to be true to self and the world. Research about childhood trauma has shown that the younger we are when traumatic events take place, the more impact the trauma will have on our future.

Before you start feeling defeated, let's be clear: We are not doomed by our past! There are many steps we can take to move forward. Unresolved trauma, however, causes problems in adult relationships. You're probably thinking something like, "I was too young to remember what happened to me or my family." While you may not remember the incident, you absorbed the impact of that trauma. Because our brain is under construction for approximately the first 25 years of life, traumatic events during childhood affect brain development AND our ability to develop healthy attachments with others. This means that each experience helps to shape your perspective and can become a lasting part of YOU—even if you can't remember the how or when of that experience. This is called a generational cycle, because there's a tendency to repeat behaviors (good or bad) that are consciously or unconsciously passed down.

Why does this matter? It matters because none of us can fully heal from the bad that occurred in our past unless we come to terms with our past—the whole truth, and nothing less.

As you unpack, you may want to seek help to explore and examine those past experiences. Although unpacking can't remove the hurt from your memories, it does position you to heal effectively, from the inside/out. In the upcoming Excursion, you'll have an opportunity to begin to unpack past experiences.

Some useful tips when unpacking:

- Don't be surprised if you find yourself repeating the same patterns that you were exposed to as a child. Our brains prefer familiarity and default to past habits until we replace them with new behaviors and information.
- Legacies and continuous cycles don't happen by chance. Instead, a pattern of behaviors can be passed along from generation to generation unless there is a break in the behavior.
- Lasting breaks in behavioral patterns typically happen by choice and not by force.

Anchors - *Takeaways*

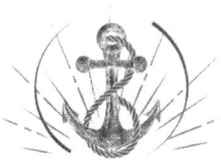

- We cannot change the past, but we CAN learn from it.
- We must be willing to examine the past in order to understand the present.
- We are products of our past; yesterday's experiences will shape tomorrow's events.
- We can choose the type of pattern/legacy we establish starting NOW.

Excursion 5 - Legacy / Patterns Activity

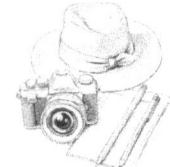

- Instructions: Give yourself some quiet time to think about the answers to the questions below.

1. What behavioral patterns/legacies can you identify in your life?

_____

_____

2. Based on your answer to Q1, which of your patterns/legacies have impacted the choices you have made recently? Last year? In the past five to 10 years? More?

_____

_____

3. Of these patterns/legacies, which do you feel are least healthy for you?

_____

_____

4. For the unhealthy patterns/legacies, what is ONE CHANGE you can commit to make which will help to break that cycle?

e.g., My dad always had a cocktail when he got home from work. I got my habit of drinking after work from him. I think if I just change that ONE THING, I could reduce the amount of alcohol I consume over the course of the week to three days instead of five.

_____

_____

5. Consider the culture (atmosphere) of your household/social circle/family. What is a pattern/legacy you may be establishing? Is it healthy or unhealthy?

_____

_____

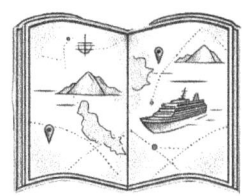 **Charter** -*Emotional Wounds*

An emotional wound is a hurt whose damage is invisible but whose presence undermines our self-esteem, self-care, mental stability, and physical well-being. Emotional pain is complex because it may have occurred recently, during childhood, or during ongoing, deliberate cruelty by an intimate partner.

The common denominator for emotional wounds is that they occur because we humans are vulnerable beings who experience a range of feelings depending on the gap between our expectations and what actually occurs. It's difficult to disappoint someone when they don't expect anything—and it's easy to hurt those who expect but don't receive. Emotional wounds, however, are NOT all the same size or depth. Like physical wounds, emotional wounds also have the potential for helping us to better understand ourselves and exercise more sound judgment in future encounters.

Types of Emotional Wounds

To be naïve is to lack experience and—as a result—the wisdom and judgment that is the product of experience. Think, for example, of learning to check a stove for heat before putting a hand near it. When we lack experience and its wisdom, we often manifest our naivete by sticking to safe and known routines. The reality is that we can reduce our naivete by partaking in life IF we are willing to risk a few scrapes, bumps, and lumps along the way. The wounds we get then build our wisdom and judgment. The catch: with each minor wound, we must apply first aid; for deeper wounds, we must seek and apply treatment.

SCRATCHES – We've all experienced disappointments that create minor detours from our intended path. Having a small set-back due to relationship conflicts is one of the most common sources of wounds. Once scratched, the injured must decide to address the issue.

How to treat NEW scratches –The best way to tend to even the tiniest paper cut is to clean it—and the same is true of emotional scratches. Like minor flesh wounds, cleaning emotional scratches requires the application of a mild antiseptic and allowing fresh air and time to facilitate organic healing. This could include talking over a disagreement after the fact, or engaging in a self-care activity like journaling about your feelings or taking a long walk.

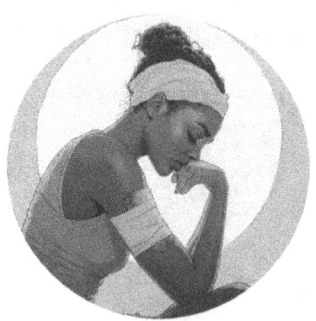

How to treat OLD scratches that have never healed – Despite being among the least life-threatening of wounds, unattended scratches tend to fester. A festering scratch attracts germs, and before long, such scratches form scabs that forever change the appearance of the skin! Negative events that happen during our youth can leave emotional scabs called trauma. The antiseptic for old sores may sting and can take some time, but it works. The antiseptic is TRUTH: being willing to face events from our past and understand why we're holding onto the event(s) is the first step. Old, unhealed scratches that have never healed might show up. An example is teasing. We might experience teasing early in life for stuttering. Although we may have outgrown the stutter, the impact of the teasing/wound can resurface in our daily interactions with others. Most of us who have OLD sores require professionals to help us face our TRUTH.

	MINOR	MAJOR
Accidental / Random	<u>Scratches</u> • Unintended • "Scratcher" may be unaware • Easy treatment • Organically healed by time and fresh air	<u>Bruises</u> • Unintended • "Bruiser" may be unaware • Treatment requires • acknowledgment of damage done, apology, and new approach • Healed by combo of self-care and atonement
Deliberate / Intimate	<u>Bites</u> • Intentional • "Bite" to coerce/control • Treatment requires atonement, conflict resolution, and re-training • Healed by combo of self-care and therapeutic intervention	<u>Breaks</u> • Intentional • "Break" to hobble, restrict, or restrain • Treatment requires atonement, conflict resolution, and re-training • Healed by combo of self-care, long-term therapy, and rehabilitation

BITES – While scratches happen accidentally, most bites are deliberate and come from someone who we have allowed to get intimately close. For these two reasons, the treatment for the emotional hurt and pain from bites is more extensive than a simple, unintentional scratch.

How to treat NEW bites – Cleaning is crucial for tending to physical bites, mainly because the mouth and teeth have germs that, once in the blood via the broken skin, can quickly get worse. An emotional bite typically requires professional support (like therapy) to ensure that the wound stays clean and free of additional damage. People are much like skin that has been damaged from a bite: vulnerable to others who might take advantage of their weakened and unprotected state. This could include scenarios like domestic violence victims who find themselves seeking companionship but who keep getting into relationships that are abusive.

How to treat OLD bruises that have yet to heal – Some bruises can do deep damage—damage that is so deep, it affects the bone. When a bone is bruised, a long period of discomfort follows. Negative impacts that go unaddressed can bleed into the surrounding muscles and cause a hard, lasting lump. Such injuries can be healed with self-care and therapy that provides the right combination of rest, elevation, compression, and possibly a topical treatment for the pain. Bad emotional bruises can also be healed with a therapeutic combination of focus on the issue, protection against further damage to the spot, and a willingness to revisit and revise how we handle the issue that has created the chronic discomfort.

BREAKS - Like bites, broken bones are often a deliberate action to restrict or control another person. If you have suffered this kind of break, you are in an unhealthy relationship and you should seek the support of someone who can help you to regain your strength to stand, walk, and run. Breaks cannot be concealed and are usually noticeable despite the injured person's attempts to discount or understate the pain. Breaks can lead to severe, long-term damage and can be crippling.

How to treat NEW breaks — While scratches and bruises build strength and character, breaks can be life-threatening; they reduce or eliminate our opportunity to apply lessons learned. The treatment includes self-care and an investment in therapy to understand how to rehabilitate our self-worth and rediscover self-reliance. Healing takes time, but the lessons learned empower us to make sounder choices for healthy relationships and better outcomes.

How to treat OLD breaks that have healed incorrectly - In movies, doctors talk about re-breaking badly set bones so the patient can heal properly. Old, deeply inflicted emotional wounds are like those bad breaks: to truly heal, they must be revisited. Like a doctor re-breaking a poorly set bone, revisiting old trauma with a professional is safer than trying to heal it on our own. With a professional, we can identify what happened, why it had the negative effects, rethink and resolve the issue, and reinvent our way of accepting the negative experience as a part of our identity.

Anchors - *Takeaways*

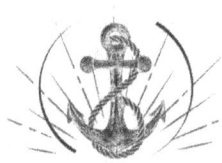

- Our emotional wounds can help strengthen our wisdom and judgment.
- Accept past hurts so they can heal.
- What doesn't kill us can indeed strengthen us!

Excursion 6 - Legacy/Patterns Activity (Wounds)

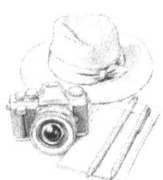

Instructions: Based on the descriptions in the prior pages:

1. Identify both a minor and a major wound you have sustained.
2. For the minor wound, think about the treatment you applied to heal it.
3. Once you've reviewed the treatment, highlight up to three personal attributes (qualities) you enhanced or strengthened as you handled the minor wound.
4. Think of how you might use those three personal attributes to begin treating (or re-treat) a MAJOR wound you sustained.
5. Using your three enhanced personal attributes, answer the questions on the next page.

What is the first action you can take to begin addressing the MAJOR wound?

_____

_____

When will you take this action?

_____

_____

Who will you include in the actions you take? Whose help will you need?

_____

_____

How will you express your need for their help?

_____

_____

Emotional Wound Selfcare

- CLEAN THE WOUND: Be honest with yourself; SEE the issue and acknowledge the damage/discomfort.
- DIAGNOSE: Identify what is actually causing the discomfort/damage.
- TREAT IT: Take action/apply the treatment and follow through.
- ACCEPT IT: Use the experience to strengthen and enhance your ability to deal with future challenges (build resiliency).

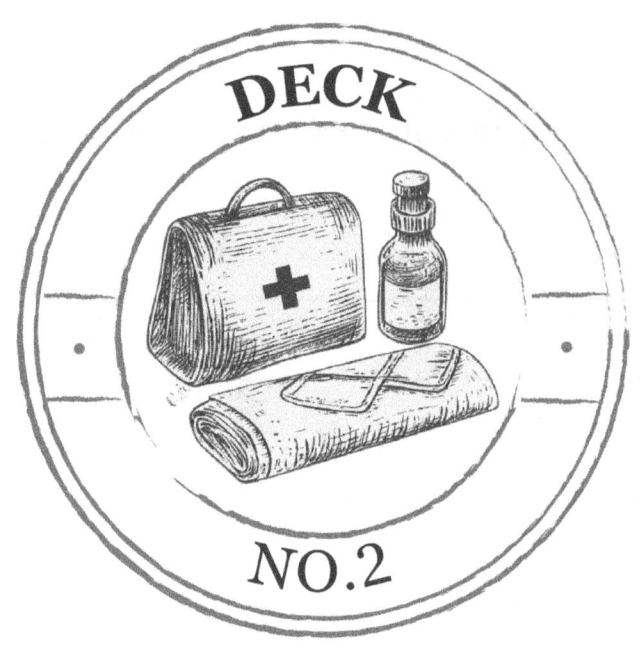

DECK 2

ACCEPT/HEAL DECK

Acceptance and Healing.

An important aspect of discovering your Authentic Self is the rediscovery of your purpose. The Accept/Heal deck facilitates the rediscovery of our purpose in life and gives meaning to the things that we experience. As we accept and heal, we get a burst of emotional energy that helps us to proceed with greater meaning and purpose. It changes how we engage in all of our relationships.

Acceptance and healing can only take place when we are aware of our hurts and have accepted that we need help. It is an ongoing pursuit and puzzle: as we get in touch with our hurts and discover ourselves, the scattered pieces of our life begin to connect and reveal our individual, unique beauty. Acceptance and healing help us review past experiences, put events in perspective, and embrace our hurt with the knowledge that it's part of our unique story. Acceptance and healing helps us tell our stories with clarity and conviction, knowing that our journey is uniquely our own.

Because we all need psychological safety, it is when we engage in healing that couples can find themselves pulling away from one another or asking for space to heal. If this is not communicated properly, our partner may interpret this need for space as an indication of disinterest as physical and/or emotional intimacy might drop. When such dynamics occur, it's important for partners to maintain open communication and demonstrate patience with one another. Each must resist the urge to rush through acceptance and healing.

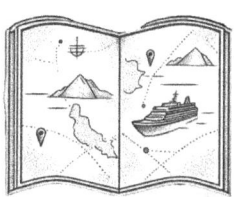 **Charter** - *Feel to Heal... Scientifically Speaking*

The human body has a natural process for handling the wounds it sustains. The four distinct stages of wound healing are:

1. Hemostasis (stop the bleeding),
2. Clotting (blood glue, plug the wound),
3. Rebuilding (create new tissue),
4. Maturation (strengthening, even if it looks healed).

Unlike body tissue, our emotional wounds may be invisible to others. What we can see on a person's outside may not reflect what's happening inside.

Many of us wear masks and pretend to be okay when we're actually torn up within. Unfortunately, wearing such masks puts us out of touch with our own condition. Most of us are ill-equipped for handling emotional wounds, so we default to unhealthy coping mechanisms like substance abuse and compulsive shopping.

Despite our traumas and coping-mechanism varying, we all have in common an internal threat response system. It dictates how we manage crises. The four general threat responses are:

- Fight
- Flight
- Freeze
- Fawn

Our internal hardwiring and life experiences determine the response to which we default. Since our bodies are wired to manage short-term stress, we may experience adverse side-effects when stress levels remain high. These side effects can be both emotional and physical as they inhibit our achieving a Healthy Me.

The discovery of our Authentic Self is neither easy nor familiar, especially upon our initial embracing of it. Our masks are carefully crafted over our lifetime and will therefore take time to remove. For example:

Ralph and Gwen were a married couple whose relationship began in high school and lasted through their early forties. It took Ralph years to embrace his Authentic Self, especially relative to Gwen's own Authentic Self and that of each of her family members who were involved in the couple's lives. Even once Ralph/Gwen were clearer on their Authentic Selves, they stayed married because so many factors made staying together seem like the easiest route. They continued working on their relationship, and Ralph began pushing Gwen to limit her time with her family, as he felt she prioritized them over him. He was surprised to discover that this had been bothering him for years, though he hadn't known himself well enough to realize that sooner.

Eventually, Ralph realized that the changes he desired of Gwen were neither fair nor realistic; they wanted different things. He asked that they divorce. Ralph learned that the journey is not quick, and it requires a huge amount of internally honest, hard work, often in personal areas that he had never previously visited.

A major effort of the healing process is to allow ourselves to move outside of our comfort zone and feel the pain. This often means revisiting traumatic experiences so we can work through the pain. As is true with physical wounds, a point comes when we must remove the emotional bandage to air the wound so it can heal properly—and when we expose wounds, we're bound to feel discomfort. Discomfort is a **healthy sign** that we have found an area that needs our attention; this attention will begin the necessary process of **working through the pain.**

There is no magic to the healing process. There is also a good chance that we will never forget the incident/event that caused the wound. All that being true: emotional wounds that are addressed will not have the same debilitating, growth-inhibiting impact.

A Healing Tool

Mindfulness is an effective tool for working through trauma and pain. It's a technique that soothes our thinking and emotions while we find new ways to manage our trauma triggers. It can include meditation, yoga, journaling, and anything else that allows us to be present and reflective. Mindfulness allows us to be in-the-moment and avoid running from our discomfort. To exercise mindfulness, we need not mentally fixate on the incident; instead, we must acknowledge it then pivot to a place we'd rather be. In some instances, exposure therapy (a component of mindfulness) is an effective tool used to reintroduce something related to the trauma in a safe environment as we then work through our fear/hurt. Mindfulness allows us to safely regulate our emotions as we go through the healing process.

Mindfulness Activity

Jon Kabat-Zinn helps us understand how mindfulness is one of the keys to healing in his book, *Coming to Our Senses: Healing Ourselves and the World Through Mindfulness*. In the book, one of the most powerful quotes to guide you is:

"Remember that the power to heal is inside of you—and so is acceptance."

Step 1 - Mindfulness. Be here, in the present moment. Don't rehash last week or anticipate the challenges of tomorrow. To do so, pick an object near you on which to focus: a lamp, a rug, etc. Find an aspect about that object that you can appreciate and begin to describe it to yourself. Be grateful for the potential being alive entails. In one of the most soul-stirring solos of the 2016 Tony award-winning musical *The Color Purple*, the main character Celie expresses the POWER of mindfulness in the lyrics of "I'm Here" that reflect her gratitude for having overcome so much abuse.

Step 2 - Gratefulness. Countless studies have proven that if we experience and express appreciation, the neurological connections in our brain are strengthened. This makes it more probable that the "feel good" chemicals will happen AGAIN. It becomes this cycle of positives rather than the proverbial vicious cycle. The more positive we are, the more positivity we attract from the environment around us.

To start, try identifying one thing you're grateful for in a journal, at the beginning of each day or end of each day.

***Anchors** - Takeaways*

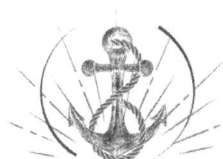

- Our pathway to healing begins when we face issues and problems.
- Facing and going through the discomfort and pain leads us to Healthy Me.
- Mindfulness is one way to begin accepting ourselves and healing

Excursion 7 - Get Started Now Activity

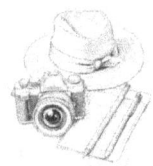

Instructions: Close your eyes. Take a few long, lung-filling, deep breaths, and then exhale them as slowly as you took them in. Try to empty your lungs when you exhale. Don't rush. Take your time. Push everything out of your mind. Everything. Pretend your mind is a blank sheet of paper.

With your eyes closed, think of a pleasant idea. Identify WHY it's so pleasant and what about it you appreciate. Think of how those positive concepts/things are having a positive impact on you and others you care about.

Stay in this mode for as long as possible—eyes closed, relaxed, and thinking of this pleasantry for which you are so very grateful.

NOTE: If you feel yourself allowing worrying thoughts to creep in, change the "pleasant" item/place/person to something else.

STOP ~ BREATHE DEEPLY/EXHALE ~ EYES CLOSED
~ PLEASANTRY ~ GRATEFULNESS ~REPEAT

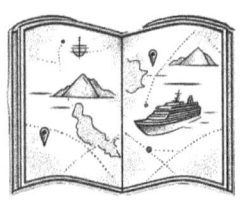

Charter - *It Takes A Village*

The African saying, "It takes a village to raise a child," is about the many influences on us as we grow into our adult selves. Much of what we learn is designed to help us first to survive and then to become, hopefully, the best version of ourselves. Yet despite these good intentions, all of us absorb more than just what is deliberately provided or shown to us. We each are shaped by a "faculty" of people: parents, siblings, extended family, teachers, coaches, friends, and many others. Some were deliberate in their methods, and others accidentally influenced us—but no matter by design or default, we were exposed to it, and influenced by it.

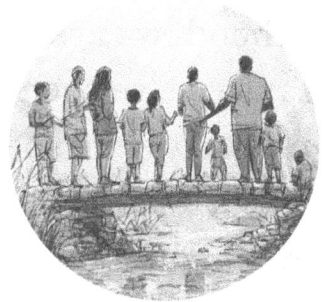

The common message our faculty provides helps us to shape our image: that head-to-toe thing we show the world, which functions as both a mask and a shield. As our faculty helps us create this mask, they emphasize its importance to our success—as if it were a device with special powers to ensure safe passage in a threatening world. The mantra, which is subtle but reinforcing, goes something like this:

**When the world looks at you, always show it_____,
and never show it _____.**

Because of that consistent message, you create an inner, shield-holding person. This is your "ALWAYS" person, the version of you who holds up your shield. Our ALWAYS person is who we show the world when the spotlight is on us or we want to be perceived as our BEST self.

But there's something else going on, something we can't avoid when the light is on: we also cast a shadow. That shadow is every bit as much a part of who we are, despite all of the work our faculty do to help us build our shield.

The shadow holds the parts of us that the faculty tell us to NEVER show. That shadow is ever-present and contains other aspects of ourselves that can provide insights, if we're brave enough to acknowledge its existence and access the wealth of information it holds.

By the time we reach adulthood, we are fully familiar with our ALWAYS person. But because we've spent so much time perfecting our ALWAYS person, we've spent little to no time gaining the insights our NEVER person can provide. None of this is surprising since we were taught to hide everything associated with our NEVER person. And the real kicker? We work extremely hard to hide our NEVER person from ourselves, too!

Here's where all of that changes. Being your Authentic Self means being completely real and honest with yourself. It means admitting that you cast a shadow—the NEVER person—and acknowledging the the shadow is also part of who you are. Maybe it starts with admitting that our village/faculty meant well; they did what they did to help us make it through the challenges they anticipated us facing. Despite their good intentions, their messages may have even been filled with words and ideas you now realize were inaccurate.

Being clear about who you are, and accepting both your ALWAYS and your NEVER person, is a perpetual quest. It requires you to take notice of behaviors that seemingly pop out from nowhere so you can determine WHY the behavior popped up. Once you know it's there, you can analyze and address that behavior.

> ***Anchors*** *- Takeaways*
>
>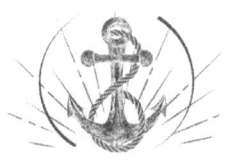
>
> - We have all been taught to keep parts of ourselves "hidden" and in the shadows.
> - Have the courage to find out what you've learned to hide, even from yourself.
> - Facing what we're hiding from can help us understand and tap potential strengths. It can reduce the barriers to living as our Authentic Self.

Excursion 8 - Lessons from Our Shadow

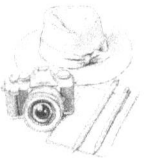

(An Activity Adapted from John Scherer's "Peeling the Onion" exercise)

We receive innumerable lessons from well-meaning members of our faculty. Their lessons are designed to help us develop the ALWAYS person we show the world. Our NEVER person, however, can also teach us lessons. Because we learned to keep these aspects of ourselves well-hidden, we may not be able to recognize our NEVER person, let alone learn from them.

Realizing that we cast a shadow is a critical step to understanding our full, Authentic Selves. The next critical step is to find the valuable information waiting for us in our NEVER person by peeling away many layers of warnings, messages, and events that reinforced our keeping it hidden.

Peeling away so many layers can stir up feelings. Be prepared for similar effects you'd get from peeling an onion: tears. It's all part of you, the AUTHENTIC you.

Excursion 8 cont. - Lessons from Our Shadow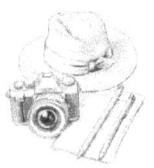

1: List below as many "ALWAYS be..." messages as you can recall. These can be direct lessons as well as indirect messages you received about how to behave when others are watching. Examples of direct messages: boys being told that only girls cry, or that you should always "clean your plate" when eating a meal. You might also have received indirect messages or lessons via observing others' behaviors. An example of an indirect message/lesson might be observing parents' behavior in social settings. Although subtle, their behavior may have contributed to the "always" message/lesson you absorbed.

_____

_____

_____

_____

2: What would the consequences be if you did not behave according to your list above? What would the world think of you?

_____

_____

_____

_____

3. Based on this analysis, list below as many items as possible that you have been taught, either directly or indirectly, to NEVER be when others are watching.

_____
_____
_____
_____

4. Select one from your "NEVER be" list that is especially clear to you. For example, you might select "Never be selfish when dealing with others." We'll explore what you choose in the next question.

_____
_____
_____
_____

Excursion 9 - Now Lets Peel The Onion

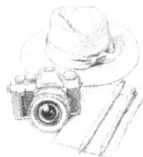

Here are three basic questions to get a deeper, closer look, using our "NEVER be selfish" example:

1. *What does a selfish person teach us? What is behind that selfishness?*

Let's say you answered: "Well, he/she is trying to beat me or win while I lose." That's probably still too negative for your "always person" to embrace.

2. *What does the selfish person need in order to win?*

Maybe we'd say "he/she needs to know what it takes to win."

3. *Would that fit on your "always be" list?*

Isn't knowing what it takes to be successful a useful, viable attribute?

Congratulations, you've just identified a positive life lesson from your shadow!

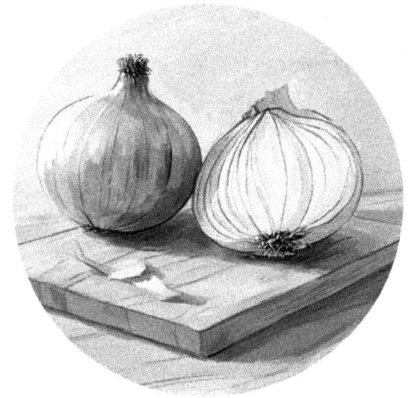

Peeling My Onion Activity

Start with the item you selected from your "never be" list.

Item: _____

1. *What is behind that item?*

_____

_____

_____

2. What must the person know or possess to achieve that outcome?

_____

_____

_____

_____

3. Would that item be useful or helpful to you, without violating your "always be" person?

_____

_____

_____

_____

When you've peeled the onion far enough, you have just allowed your "never be" person to teach you to be more complete. Our shadow is with us all the time. It is a part of us and, if we let it, it can help us move toward (and gain comfort in living as more of our Authentic Self.).

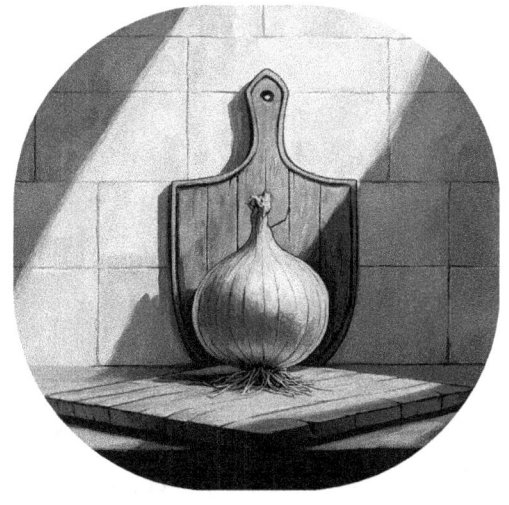

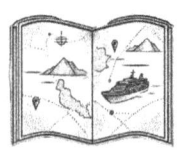 **Charter** - *Forgiveness: The Untapped Superpower*

FORGIVENESS (noun): a conscious, deliberate decision to release feelings of resentment or vengeance toward a person or group who has harmed you, regardless of whether they deserve that release or not.

~adapted from Psychology Today

When you examine forgiveness, it's clear why it can be so difficult to practice: it requires us to LET GO. We must let go of what's familiar, what may have been with us for a long time, and what could drastically change the routines to which we've grown accustomed. On top of that, it may also require us to let go of strong—and valid—emotions like anger, blame, resentment, etc. Letting go of these is particularly difficult, as withholding forgiveness keeps you emotionally connected to a group or person. This means you're not only letting go of feelings you're used to, but you're also letting go of that connection, too. In addition to the connection, by withholding forgiveness we can often feel the added bonus of wielding punishment THAT WE CONTROL. Forgiveness asks us to let go of that, too.

Despite such seemingly powerful potential to crush our perceived enemies, withholding forgiveness is actually like holding onto a live wire: it hurts the one holding it. The longer you hold on, the more damaged you'll be.

How can that be? To understand it better, consider whatever grievance you have and whomever you have it with THE ISSUE. Imagine THE ISSUE is the shape of a cat, looks like a cat, has teeth and claws like a cat, and makes hissing sounds like a cat. You are carrying around and feeding THE ISSUE. Each time you allow yourself to think about THE ISSUE, you feel like you're being scratched by its thin, razor-sharp claws. Yet you persist.

There are even some days the annoyance gets so intense; the scratch feels more like several bites into your hands and arms. As cat bites often do, yours get infected and cause severe swelling. You know you're going to need medical attention, but you keep carrying THE ISSUE. What would happen if you released it?

When you release THE ISSUE, it is no longer close enough to inflict damage. THE ISSUE either resolves itself (imagine a cat that walks away) or sidles up to you to demonstrate a desire to reconnect without being carried (imagine a cat that purrs for attention). Once THE ISSUE has been released, you can move freely; both of your hands can address your own needs, wounds, and work. This is how FORGIVENESS feels—like releasing a ball of constant energy that is wreaking havoc on your body. Emancipation. Freedom from the chore of carrying negative energy.

Just what are you doing when you forgive? You're gifting yourself more time and energy for what truly matters. You're freeing mental real estate that can be used for positive construction projects like new friends, new love, new interests, etc.

You're probably thinking, "It can't be that simple—nothing is that easy." You're right. There are two important rules to remember about forgiveness to help you muscle through the challenge:

1. It is INTENTIONAL. You grant freedom to YOURSELF.
2. The forgiven need never know. It's not about them; it's YOURS TO GIVE YOURSELF. If the forgiven are still alive/available and continue to have access to you, the only thing they may notice is your newly-minted peacefulness and tranquility.

If I forgive, must I FORGET? And other puzzling questions

There are other sides to forgiveness that make letting go difficult. Examples include situations of betrayal and/or when the ISSUE is the result of someone else's behavior—particularly someone else's HABITUAL, recurring behavior. Simple psychology tells us that if a person experiences an advantage by behaving badly, they will do it again. How can we forgive when that happens?

The answer is a bit more complex than simply releasing the cat (by letting go). If a bad behavior persists, we may need a few preliminary steps if we are to truly forgive—starting with confronting the person. This assumes, of course, the person is available. If so, the preliminary steps are ones commonly used to resolve conflict and begin with giving the other person feedback. If the mutual understanding that results from the conversation doesn't create the mental space and opportunity for you to then "let go" and forgive, it's time for more extreme measures; these would likely include limiting the other person's access to you so no further harm can occur. If after exercising self-care/self-preservation measures we can forgive, even if the behavior happens again, we are much less vulnerable and very likely impervious to their bad behavior. The perpetrators are left "shadowboxing."

Just forgiving another person does not give them license to continue to hurt us. Forgiveness is a choice we make for ourselves. Another positive by-product of having that difficult discussion from a place of forgiveness is that it can benefit the relationship. Such conversations can strengthen the connection between you and the other person. At a minimum, it brings truth and honesty to the relationship. Returning to our cat analogy, the honest discussions keep the cat close by, but with warmth and understanding. Forgiveness makes a space to release grudges and negativity. Here's an example:

Pete was thrilled to finally find Tom, a reliable tenant for the apartment attached to his house. One of the most attractive aspects of Tom's situation was that he was multi-skilled and motivated to repair things when they needed it or work outside on landscaping. Pete and Tom reached a compensation agreement for the work Tom completed. In a short time, Pete and Tom became friends.

Their friendship hit a significant obstacle when Tom hurriedly back his truck down the driveway and ran over Pete's son's bicycle, mangling it beyond repair. The part of this event that hurt Pete the most was that Tom had little or no remorse; Tom was content to blame the tragedy on the little boy for leaving the bike on the driveway.

Eventually, Pete came to realize that each person's explanation stemmed from their own unique perspective. Pete began to let go of the discomfort he felt with Tom's attitude about the bike. He felt no need to discuss his attitude shift with Tom, but he did feel that he needed one conversation with Tom to ask that Tom check behind the truck for safety reasons when backing out—and Tom agreed immediately.

Once Pete let go of his own emotional reactions, he realized that his reactions were based on his perceptions and he was empowered to change them.

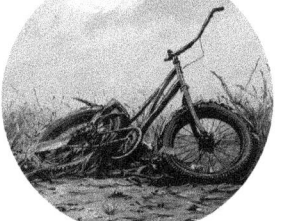

Anchors - Takeaways

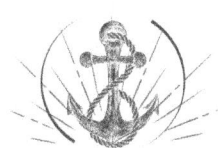

- Forgiveness is about letting go.
- It's not necessary to inform those who have been forgiven because forgiveness is something you do for YOUR WELL-BEING.
- We don't forgive because we want to free others; we forgive to free ourselves.

Excursion 10 - The Art of Forgiving

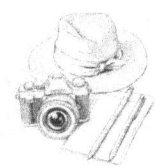

Find a Source:

Identify someone who has wronged you in the past. This may be a person with whom you have talked out the disagreement, or it may be someone who has no idea how you feel.

My Target to Forgive _____

How does this person enrich your life

_____
_____
_____
_____

How is this person an obstacle or roadblock in your life?

_____
_____
_____
_____

What will it take for you to forgive this person thoroughly and completely?

_____

_____

_____

_____

Remember: Once this act is forgiven, it should not require further discussion. You can decide whether or not you'll tell the other person about your act of forgiveness. The act of forgiving is FOR YOU and you do not need anyone else's permission.

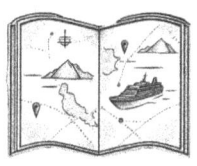 **Charter** - *Letting Go*

A major component to healing is letting go of the self-constructed barriers to a Healthy Me. Letting go means we understand that we can't change others. This includes friends, family, and partners—we can't save them. Every partner, be they an intimate partner or platonic friend, joins you either temporarily or long-term. When we must let go of relationships, it need not mean that we don't care; instead, it means that we must care for ourselves and take responsibility for our choices instead of trying to save or change them.

Letting go also means we can process and release past feelings and hurts. With such a release we can accept that every experience puts us more in touch with our Authentic Self. Letting go brings each of us closer to our Healthy Me. The freedom that results from letting go allows us to choose to see the good in every experience, removes fear and anxiety from our response to difficulties, and compels us to embrace the challenge of learning from our experiences.

Sky lanterns are used for many reasons. Many people use them in ceremonies that fill the night sky with a sea of individual lights; each light represents a burdensome concern like a chronic illness or an ongoing challenge. Regardless of the symbolic meaning behind each lantern, the one common action for those who partake in such a ceremony is TO RELEASE THE LANTERN.

Imagine attending a wedding and refusing to let go of the hand of the person with whom you walked down the aisle; or, as a parent on the first day of kindergarten, holding onto your child throughout the day. Seen from this angle, holding on seems preposterous because there are adventures and growth awaiting the member of the wedding or that eager young mind!

So why do we hold onto people, anger, situations, past transgressions, etc.? Despite our knowing deep down that—like the flame within the sky lantern—holding on allows the flame to continually burn us? The wisdom of this adage is a clear call to action:

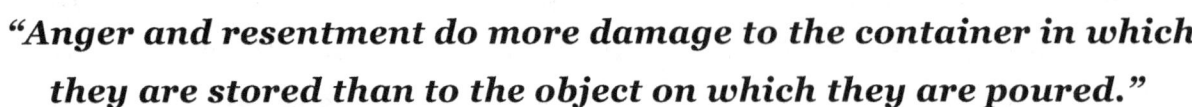

"Anger and resentment do more damage to the container in which they are stored than to the object on which they are poured."

" ~Adapted from Mark Twain

Excursion 11- Letting Go Activity

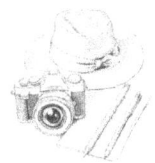

1. Identify at least three events in your life story when you successfully let go of someone or something important to you. These would be those moments when your heart says to hang on, but your brain knows letting go is the right thing to do.

Example: Letting go of your five-year-old-child on the first day of school.

_____

_____

_____

_____

2. Choose one scenario from your list. What were positive results of that "letting go" for you and/or the person you released?

_____

_____

_____

_____

_____

_____

3. What would have been the consequences if you had not been able to let go?

_____

_____

_____

FORMULA FOR LETTING GO/HEALING:

Awareness + Acknowledgement + Releasing Negative Feelings

Awareness & Acknowledgement

If you've never looked into a mirror, then you truly haven't built self-awareness. You don't necessarily need to look into a literal mirror, as self-awareness is a mirror of its own. The many mirrors available to give you awareness can be found in the feedback of loved ones, situations that have gone wrong, and relationships filled with mistakes. To be a fully effective and potent ingredient for healing, awareness must be accompanied by acknowledgement.

For a simple example of the effectiveness of awareness and acknowledgement, we need only recall those typical times that we've accidentally stepped on someone's toe while waiting in a queue. When we realize our mistake and utter a sincere acknowledgment and apology, we typically find the matter ended. Awareness AND acknowledgment allow negative feelings to evaporate.

For an example of awareness without acknowledgement, picture the same scenario: You step on someone's toe, they tell you, and you ignore them, neither acknowledging the action nor gaining any insight regarding the location of your feet in relation to someone else's feet!

In the latter foot-stepping incident, the healing of the bruised foot/feelings is postponed and replaced (potentially) by an escalation of anger—on the part of both parties. The longer the awareness and acknowledgment are delayed, the less likely it is that healing will occur. Each person may have missed out on what might have been a terrific friendship, companionship, or other REALationship. What's even more certain: each will typically carry the negativity of that event into subsequent interactions they have with others, never realizing the power they each have for creating more space in their lives for happiness. When it comes to stepping on someone's toe, the effects don't linger long, but when it comes to betrayal or deliberate cruelty, the effects are much more serious.

To many people, the act of releasing feels like a loss. Yet when we consider the following parable of a wise elder speaking to a brash youth, we can better understand the enormous strength we gain within ourselves by actually letting go:

Brash Youth: "Please, Elder, tell me the most important things you've learned so that I may take a shortcut to a successful future."

Wise Elder: "Fill this bucket and this glass with water from the river and set them before me."

The Brash Youth does as he is instructed. Then, his voice filled with impatience, he says to Wise Elder, "I'm anxious and ready for the shortcut, please tell me."

Wise Elder: "Fill the glass with water from the bucket."

Brash Youth: "You know the glass is already full and it can hold no additional water. Why do you taunt and delay?"

Wise Elder: "You are the glass, and I am the bucket. I can only give you what is available from me when you release what you are holding."

Moral of the story: Be willing to let go so that you can grow

So why do we hold on? The answers are many and complex, but most boil down to a simple truth: we've never given ourselves a chance to practice letting go. In the next few pages, we'll provide ways for you to re-examine the barriers associated with release. By the end of this topic, you'll gain insights on how letting go helps you purge negative past events so you can free yourself to grab the positive, bright future that lies ahead of you!

*Examples of Barriers to Letting Go**

> Blaming Others - Holding Resentment - Guilt - Unforgiveness

*NOTE: If you feel ANY of the above barriers, you're ready to find your strength and feel the power of letting go.

CONSIDERATIONS That Raise SELF-AWARENESS

CONSIDER: If you are resentful about what someone else did or continues to do, that person is controlling your feelings. That person is still able to make you feel bad.

> *Explore for Self-Awareness:* Do you want this person to be able to control how you feel?

> *Explore for Self-Awareness:* What do you believe about the "CONSIDER" statement and how is it relevant for you?

CONSIDER: In some ways, getting angry or resenting someone is like taking poison and waiting for someone else to die.

> *Explore for Self-Awareness:* What do you believe about this statement and how is it relevant for you?

CONSIDER: To forgive means to pardon. To pardon means to release from punishment. If you pardon a guilty person, it does not excuse the person for his crimes or suggest they did not occur. It only means that continued punishment is not worth the energy and cost that would be required.

> *Explore for Self-Awareness:* Do you want to spend the rest of your life as, for example, your ex-partner's jailer or warden? What kind of life would that be?

CONSIDER: Holding onto anger is like putting on your daily TO DO LIST "Spend time being angry."

> *Explore for Self-Awareness:* Will getting angry improve your day or your future? Can you take it off of your TO DO LIST?

CONSIDER: Letting go of anger simply requires a decision. Anger requires rumination. Anger requires a memory or thought about unfair treatment, often accompanied by thoughts of wanting to hurt someone or see them suffer. In other words, anger is a CHOICE, and your anger is controllable. You can choose to stop being angry.

> *Explore for Self-Awareness:* Will you break the anger habit by making a decision to stop obsessing about unfairness? Can you change the subject, which is taking up so much real estate in your mind? How is this relevant for you?

CONSIDER: Immediately after asking why you or a loved one has been treated unfairly, ask yourself the second question: What will I do about it? If the answer is, "I'm not going to do anything to improve the situation," whatever else you do is a time waster. If there are no satisfying answers to the question, you should at LEAST decide to stop obsessing in a way that makes you feel bad. Sometimes what happened, though tragic and undeserved, may have just been poor luck.

> *Explore for Self-Awareness:* What do you believe about this statement and how is it relevant for you?

CONSIDER: Are any of the following among your favorite ways to curse the darkness?

- *There is no justice!*
- *It's not fair.*
- *I was set up/deceived.*
- *How dare he/she?*
- *How could anyone be so cruel?*
- *Why would someone do something like that?*
- *It never should have happened!*
- *That [expletive]!*
- *I hate their guts. I hope they rot in hell!*

Do you actually ever feel better by yelling such comments? Probably not—or, if so, just temporarily. Emotionally charged words never solve anything. When thinking about an injustice, you'll feel better if you use neutral or descriptive words rather than emotionally charged or derogatory ones.

Explore for Self-Awareness: What do you believe about this statement, and how is it relevant for you?

CONSIDER: Anger expressed toward someone who is the source of your frustration neither increases the chances of that person giving you what you want nor stops the behavior you dislike. Expressing anger usually escalates conflict and alienates the person who is the target of your anger.

Explore for Self-Awareness: The next time you hear yourself saying or thinking, I'm angry... mad.... pissed off... resentful, change your words to: I'm frustrated, or I'm upset, or my feelings are hurt. Angry people fight, say things that are hurtful, demonstrate hostility, or are just plain mean, but they rarely solve problems. Frustrated people, on the other hand, focus on the obstacle or problem that is the source of the frustration; THAT activates problem-solving.

Explore for Self-Awareness: What do you believe about this statement and how is it relevant for you?

CONSIDER: Getting angry at someone who isn't even present is the ultimate act of futility. It's like having a prizefight with yourself; you always lose.

Explore for Self-Awareness: What do you believe about this statement and how is it relevant for you?

CONSIDER: Engage in the following 'Releasing the Other Person' Activity:

- *List all the things she/he did to you.*
- *List all the things you did to her/him.*
- *Ball up the list and toss it in the trash. You can't make other people change or force others to be accountable for their behaviors.*

Explore for Self-Awareness: Each day, make one list of the benefits of letting go, and another of the consequences of holding on. What do you notice about your lists?

Anchors - *Takeaways*

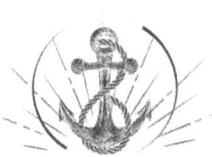

- Letting go helps us purge the negative past and leaves us free to grab the positive future!
- Awareness AND acknowledgment allow negative feelings to evaporate, leaving room for a conversation.
- Be willing to let go so you can grow.

Excursion 11A- Letting Go Activity

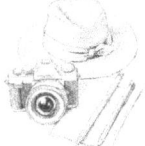

(REMEMBER: Forgiveness is the emotional de-cluttering you do to free up space, time, and energy—for yourself.)

Getting Started : This is typically the hardest part. Take inventory by answering these questions:

- *What happened?*
- *Who was involved?*
- *How were you impacted?*
- *Why do you still remember it?*
- *How is it affecting you today?*

Gaining Momentum : Give yourself a positive vision. Imagine your life if the issue/person/people no longer entered your thoughts.

- *How might you spend your time?*
- *How would you organize your space?*
- *What would your energy level be? (e.g., low, moderate, high)*

Soar: Try letting go. See if you experience the feeling of freedom created by your choices. It may take some time—a week, a month, or more. Whatever the time lapse, try to describe the positive impact your choice to let go/forgive has had in these areas:

- *Sleep*
- *Appetite*
- *Fitness*
- *Physical Comfort*
- *Interests*
- *Friends*
- *Family*
- *Home life*
- *Work life*

To get the best results, try starting with small acts of letting go. What's small for you may be huge for others, so you decide. The most important thing is to start. With practice we make progress.

Excursion 11B - Identifying Healing Points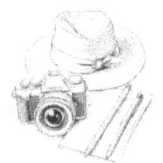

Instructions: **Return to your T3 Assessment** in the **Explore Deck (Page 66)** to identify areas of your life that still need to be addressed. These areas that are still in need are called healing points. For example, your T3 might indicate a healing point around someone who hurt you or resentment you may still feel towards a friend.

In the next Charter, you'll learn more about ways of addressing those healing points which will ultimately lead to acceptance.

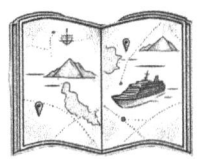 **Charter** - *Acceptance Leads to Healing*

Acceptance is about facing and acknowledging the objective truth; as such, acceptance is a critical part of healing. Although it's natural to want to distance ourselves from uncomfortable or bad experiences, stalling, avoiding, or ignoring pain significantly delays our healing. Think about what healing really means: "to make whole again." To begin examining your own healing, consider the following questions:

4 Questions to Get Started

1. Do you repel memories and avoid aspects of your life that have caused you significant hurt?
2. Do you justify being hurt by someone you love and, ultimately, choose to give them a pass so you'll feel better about ignoring their poor treatment of you?
3. Do you ignore the trauma you've sustained from bad encounters, choosing instead to exaggerate the positives?
4. Do you revise your childhood or relationships to be more pleasant or satisfying

NOTE: If you answered YES to any of the four questions, you are actively hindering your own healing.

A symptom is the body's way of letting us know that something needs attention. When we separate ourselves from, ignore, or fail to acknowledge our symptoms, we do the exact opposite of healing. Healing is made possible when we choose to stop resisting and denying what is happening and start accepting the fact: Something IS happening, and it IS painful/hurtful.

When we begin to accept the pain (or any symptom we're experiencing), the healing process can begin because we are no longer mentally cutting ourselves off from the experience; instead, we're allowing the energy to be released and to flow through—and eventually OUT of our body.

Keep in mind that acceptance neither equates to liking the situation nor surrendering to it. Acceptance simply means we are no longer resisting it. Accepting facts neither minimizes their significance nor our feelings about them. Acceptance is the first step in the process of healing.

"We cannot fix what we won't face." ~James Baldwin

Imagine: your best friend is a three-pack-a-day smoker. No matter how concerned you are, the only control you have are your words and deeds. You can't stop them from smoking, but you can help or hinder the healthy choices made by your friend. If you fully accept the facts and let go of what is out of your control, you are freed-up to do MORE in areas where you have control—your words and deeds. Positive psychology helps us maximize life experiences by understanding the sources of happiness and ways people thrive. To benefit most from positive psychology, we must learn to accept that there are limits to our personal control:

WE are the ONLY thing we can control. Accepting that fact is where we must start if we want to get the most out of life.

We've said much about what acceptance isn't; now let's explore more about what acceptance IS and how it changes our lives for the better.

Part of why we benefit from acceptance is the strength and resiliency it allows us to manifest. Research has proven that our willingness to accept the unchangeable contributes mightily to our emotional and psychological well-being. There is no better example of fortitude than working through a situation that seemed unsurmountable. Making it through a period of depression, enduring a difficult labor to deliver a baby, and/or struggling to pay off a mountain of financial debt are all examples of actions that, once completed, help us feel especially relieved AND accomplished. Most people express enormous pride that they've gained first-hand proof about the timeless adage: What doesn't break you makes you stronger! We emerge from such experiences with a greater understanding of ourselves and our personal strengths, as well as increased knowledge of how to avoid such pitfalls and (possibly most important of all) self-respect. Self-respect is core to emotional and psychological well-being.

In the 1994 blockbuster movie The Shawshank Redemption, one of the central characters, embodies the concept of maintaining emotional and psychological well-being despite experiencing countless atrocities at the penitentiary. Describing the protagonist, his friend and confidante said, "It goes back to what I said about [him]wearing his freedom like an invisibility coat, about how he never really developed a prison mentality. His eyes never got that dull look." The protagonist realized that although prison is a brick-and-mortar location designed to eliminate any sense of self-agency (control) for inmates, the experience couldn't take from him what he'd already established: a love of beauty, his desire to learn, helping others appreciate life's beauty, and his amazing accounting skills. That character said, "There are places in this world that aren't made out of stone. That there's something inside...that they can't get to, that they can't touch. That's yours." Finally, and determined to prevail in a situation that seemed insurmountable, the protagonist tells his friend: "I guess it comes down to a simple choice really. Get busy living or get busy dying."

The protagonist accepted the reality of prison. To long for it to be something it wasn't would be the very definition of lack of acceptance. His acceptance fueled his 20-year prison-break project. The Rienhold Niebuhr prayer that has been popularized by Alcoholics Anonymous might have even served as a type of mantra for the character:

"God, grant me the serenity to accept the things I cannot change, the courage to change the things I can, and the wisdom to know the difference."

Acceptance allowed the character to rebound from the many setbacks he experienced, continue to use his skills to create foolproof action plans, and maintain ever-readiness to execute his plan when the opportunity surfaced. While he didn't heal within the confines of the penitentiary, he never succumbed to its horrors. He maintained emotional and psychological well-being that enabled him to break free to the locale where his long and redemptive healing could take place.

> **Anchors - *Takeaways***
>
>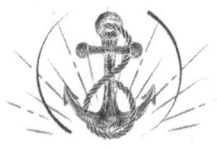
> - Acceptance is the first step in the healing process.
> - We benefit from acceptance because it demonstrates our strength and resiliency while building self-respect.
> - Self-respect is core to emotional and psychological well-being.

Excursion 12 - How to Get Busy Healing

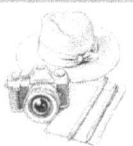

Let's repeat our earlier mindfulness activity, this time applying it to acceptance. Remember that the power to heal is inside of you—and so is acceptance.

1. Mindfulness. Be here, in the present moment. Don't rehash last week or anticipate the challenges of tomorrow. Be HERE. For example, try to focus on just one item in the room. Once you have fixated on it, start to describe it for yourself. Take in as many details as you can—what do you see? Express gratitude for what you are taking in via your senses.

2. Countless studies have proven that if we experience and express appreciation, something in our brain gets strengthened. The neurological connections that happen make it more probable that the "feel good" mood that comes from doing so makes it more likely that the positives will happen again. The more positive we are, the more positivity we attract from the environment around us.

Try starting a gratitude journal which is like a diary—a diary into which you write as often as possible. Try to start each day with an entry into your gratitude journal; write down one thing you're grateful for each day. Since most of us have a notetaking function in our cell phones, try capturing your gratitude using your cell phone! Your statement doesn't have to be a long one. Here's an example: "I'm grateful for waking up this morning to a sunny day. It's been so cloudy lately, the sun made me feel really good!"

Get Started Now

Close your eyes. Take a few long, lung-filling, deep breaths and exhale them slowly. Try to empty your lungs when you exhale. Take your time.
Push everything out of your mind. Everything. Pretend your mind is a blank sheet of paper.

With your eyes closed, think of the most pleasant idea you can. Identify WHY it's so pleasant and what about it you appreciate. Think of how those positive concepts/things are having a positive impact on you and others you care about.

Stay in this mode for as long as possible—eyes closed, relaxed, and thinking of this pleasantry for which you are so very grateful.

> *NOTE: If you feel yourself allowing worrying thoughts to creep in, change the "pleasant" item/place/person to something else.*

Stop~ Breath Deeply & Exhale ~Eyes Closed~ Pleasantry~ Gratefulness ~ Repeat

---

Excursion 13- Acceptance Activity for Self Care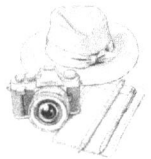

Over the next five days, begin developing your powerful potential to forgive. Use the day-corresponding questions below to help you develop the empowering habit of forgiveness and be set free.

DAY	AGREEMENT RATING
DAY 1	• Who is consuming time/space/energy in your mind? • What's making it so difficult for you to let go of it? • Is there a small part of what happened that you can forgive or let go?
DAY 2	• Say aloud and/or to yourself: "I forgive [name(s)] for [behavior/deed] throughout the day to begin creating the habit of forgiveness. Where the mind goes the body follows!" Repeat this act several times throughout the day.
DAY 3	• What is the most despicable thing that has been done to you? • Now imagine that those who did it were TAUGHT to behave that way. That's right; envision the person(s) who hurt you—see them in your mind. But this time, see them as VICTIM of someone else's meanness, abuse, etc. See them as if they were still that little, innocent child being given terrible social skills and instruction. • Envision the pain they carry. Think about the power you have to end the cycle of pain. All you need to do is side-step the negative energy; don't claim it! It started with another person long ago, but it ends with YOU.
DAY 4	• With your newfound perspective of the other person(s) as a VICTIM, start asking yourself questions like: What strengths do I exhibit when I see the perpetrator as the victim of bad instructions? • If the person(s) is still living/available, what positive attributes do they have? • Are those attributes ones that you'd like to emulate? If yes, can you shift this relationship to center around those positive attributes ONLY? • If not, can you use your understanding of these relationship challenges to help others benefit from the lessons you've learned (e.g., to coach others)?

DAY 5	<ul><li>Think about someone you have forgiven.</li><li>How did it benefit you?</li><li>How did you use the experience to help yourself? Others</li></ul>

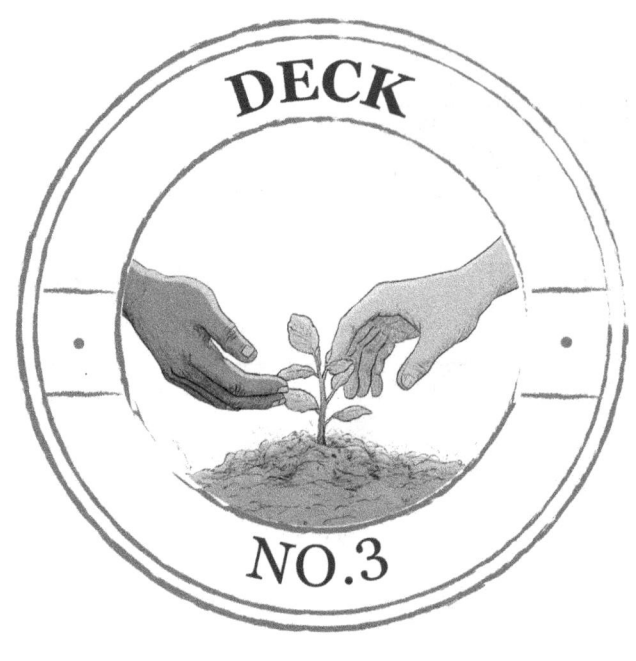

DECK 3

GROW DECK

GROWTH is a natural process. When we plant seeds in fertile soil, expose them to sunlight, and provide water—what happens is growth. Like plants, people each have a distinct growth pattern. In our model, the fertile soil, sun, and water are the personal work we do on the Explore and Heal/Accept decks. This ongoing work positions us to lean into our Authentic Self.

As is true of any garden or field of crops, weeds and overgrowth can overtake plants and choke out the sun. Like plants, people face challenges and setbacks that act as obstacles to our growth. We must expect this and continue to strive to know and embrace our Authentic Self. The more healing/acceptance we accomplish, the healthier our manifested behaviors and choices will be. In this manner, Heal/Accept/Grow are all complements to one another; there is no sustained growth without acceptance/healing.

Since growth is an ongoing pursuit, here are 10 facts, mindsets, conditions, and questions that can help us maintain our momentum over time:

FACT: We need not announce that we are growing. Others will recognize it without our pointing it out.

FACT: There is no sustained growth without healing. Healing helps us discover/re-discover our purpose and voice, both of which are critical for establishing our own goals and direction.

CONDITION: Giving up one's own goals to make others happy is a misstep that typically results from lacking one's own goals/direction; instead, the person aligns with their partner's goals and direction.

QUESTION: Do you deny your own needs just to hold onto another person? Has that resulted in you losing your sense of SELF?

FACT: Compromise and planning to support mutual goals in a relationship should not result in you losing your identity.

FACT: Continuous progress and growth allow us to remove the limits we place on ourselves.

CONDITION: Confidently share your goals/plans without expecting others to endorse them.

FACT: Healthy REALationships can only exist in an environment where each person can be themselves without feeling threatened or intimidated.

Question: Do I root for the other people in my life to win and embrace their Authentic Selves?

FACT: Growth requires us to work from inside ourselves. We seek, examine, and address ourselves from the inside out.

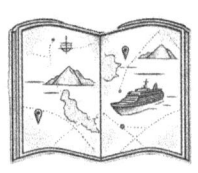 **Charter** - *Supersize My Words*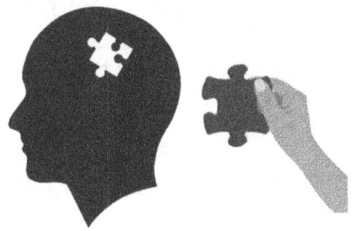

Self-talk is powerful. It's the most powerful internal conversation because where the mind goes, the body follows. It can be either positive and enabling—much like vitamins that fortify your body—or it can be negative and limiting, like a slow-acting poison. Because of its potential, positive self-talk is an effective tool available to anyone who seeks success. Self-talk acts to frame the events that happen; when events are framed positively, it helps you to sustain the progress you make toward goal achievement. Building the habit of positive self-talk is sound preparation and application for the journey toward a healthy Authentic Self.

Negative self-talk did not originate with you—some of it was placed in your mind long before you realized you could choose to block it out. Consider each thought as a piece of a puzzle. For example, as a child, maybe a respected adult said something like, "You're so clumsy," every time you made a mistake. That comment was a puzzle piece; as an adult, whenever you make a mistake, you may repeat that negative comment as self-talk.

Here's the good news: every puzzle piece/negative comment can be replaced with a positive one of your choice! This isn't about lying to ourselves; we aren't going to tell ourselves that we're ten feet tall when that isn't true. Instead, it's about choosing not to believe negative opinions which aren't facts. You can create new comments or mantras to repeat to yourself, which you can use as positive self-talk. A mantra is a word or phrase that we repeat to ourselves to override negative self-talk.

An example of this tug-of-war between positive and negative self-talk is often evident when people speak about their body. The view they have of themselves was well established in their childhood and typically those messages came from trusted others.

> *Consider Shirley, who was called "Stick" as a child and teen because her body did not develop at the same pace as her peers. Shirley's self-talk was almost completely negative because that was all she'd ever heard about herself: She believed she should have more curves like her peers.*
>
> *Through persistence and careful work as an adult, Shirley began to reconstruct those childhood messages. As she did so, Shirley realized that in addition to being thin-framed, she was ALSO musically gifted, a great athlete, and a loving, devoted family member!*
>
> *Had Shirley been able to focus on those positive aspects of herself while she developed from child through young adult, her ability to achieve loving relationships with others would likely have occurred much sooner in her life. She didn't need to worry about her body shape, because that was irrelevant in many aspects of her life. She could spend that energy elsewhere instead.*
>
> *Shirley realized that had she not done the important work of seeing the positives, she would have been locked in a prison of negative self-talk as an adult, too.*

> **Anchors** - *Takeaways*
>
>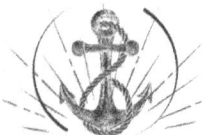
> - Self-talk is a powerful tool that can help us make progress when it's positive.
> - Mantras are positive self-talk that counteract our negative self-talk and help us develop more positive habits!

Excursion 14 - My Mantra & Antidote Activity

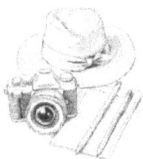

To convert negative self-talk into positive, it's important to be honest about our self-talk habits. Since most of us engage in some amount of negative self-talk, we must first conduct an INVENTORY of our typical self-talk then replace it. To do so, follow this approach:

1. List some of your typical negative self-talk. This could include:
- *I'll never amount to anything.*
- *I'm unlucky in love.*
- *I don't deserve nice things.*
- *I'm too clumsy to learn a sport.*

_____

_____

_____

_____

2. Use your list to create new mantras.
- For each of your negative self-talk items, think of a true, positive statement. This can take time and several attempts since negative self-talk often slows our ability to overcome clouded thinking and powerlessness. You may also feel like you're being fake or awkward or bragging about yourself as you begin to try to develop this behavior. Stick with it! You're undoing years and years of habit.

Recall the activity when you were "Peeling the Onion" to establish true statements about yourself—it takes time and effort. Know that you can always return to this activity to get better and better at this behavior.

To begin developing the habit of converting your negative self-talk to positive mantras, use the approach below. NOTE: Keep working until you have established a positive antidote (new mantra) to the poison of each negative self-talk comment. Here's an example:

My Negative Self-Talk: *"I'll never amount to anything."*
1st positive statement I tell myself: *"I may not have accomplished what I'd like to, but I'm still a good person."*
I then build on that more positive thought to come up with another positive thought:
2nd positive statement I tell myself: *"A good person strives to acknowledge the goodness in others AND themselves."*
I then find something even more positive to build onto my 2nd statement:

3rd positive statement I tell myself: *"My goodness is manifested whenever I'm kind to others—even when that person is someone I don't know."*
I then find something positive to build onto my 3rd statement:

4th positive statement I tell myself: *"Even if my only contribution to the world is being and bringing kindness to others, I will have achieved something!"*
I'm now ready to construct a mantra that I can repeat to myself whenever I hear myself saying "I'll never amount to anything." That mantra is:

My Mantra Antidote: *"I am a kind person, and acts of kindness are important contributions that can lead to personal achievements like happiness and self-respect."*

Now, Try It Yourself!

1. Using one of the negative self-talk phrases/statements you generated at the beginning of this excursion, try to create 3-4 positive statements like in the example. If you didn't generate any negative statements, use one of the samples provided below:

_____

_____

_____

_____

SAMPLE PHRASES:

1) I take too much time to decide things.
2) If I take a calculated risk, something bad will likely happen.
3) I shouldn't spend money on things I don't really need.
4) I didn't really like that [fill in the blank] but I'll say I did when asked.
5) Why am I spending my time doing this?
6) Why can't I just do what I was asked to do?
7) I keep harping on it.
8) If I can't do it, they'll get somebody who will.

2. Once you have made at least four attempts to build a positive statement from the original negative statement, create a mantra antidote that you can commit to memory and use

_____

_____

_____

_____

REFLECTION: Think of the phrases you hear from someone with whom you currently live, work, or consistently interact. Identify one (1) phrase that you realize you've incorporated into your own negative self-talk. Create another mantra antidote for this self-talk.

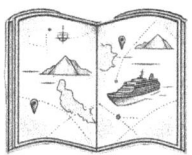

Charter - *My Growth & Progress*

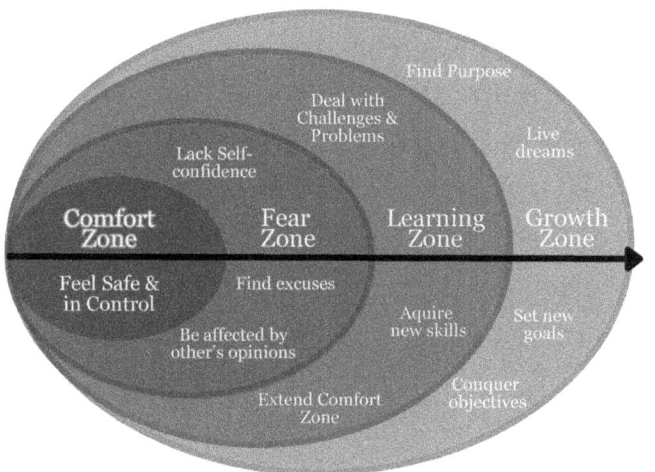

Your journey begins when you're born. In the illustration to the left, there are four zones which we experience over the course of our lives: comfort, fear, learning, and growth.

Through the illustration is a dark arrow to suggest the optimal direction in which we move throughout our lives: from comfort through growth, with fear and learning happening along the way. Most of us want our journey to be like that straight line: we want life to be simple and straightforward.

Now, imagine life's journey to be more like the illustration on the right: a trek that winds, re-visits, stalls, and re-starts, but is ever-moving. That's what life is typically like—a journey that allows us to grow only if we depart from what is comfortable, face our fears, and learn from our inevitable mistakes. Growth is what awaits us when we're willing to let go of what's comfortable. But how do we measure whether what's happening to us has resulted in actual growth? Do we have gauges or measuring sticks for emotional growth the way we did as kids, measuring our physical height against a wall or doorframe? The answer: we each have a gauge tailored to measure our unique, personal growth—IT RESIDES WITHIN US.

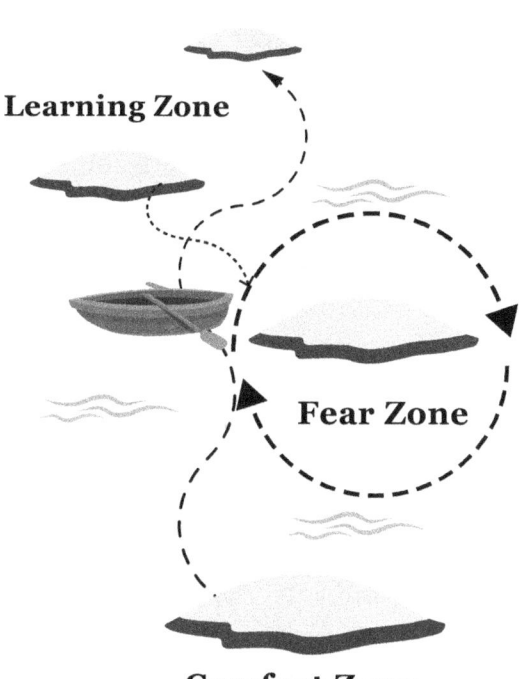

WARNING: The adage about how comparing yourself to others causes unhappiness is especially true. In childhood some of us marked our physical growth using pencil marks on a doorframe, which conditioned us to look for growth via visible comparison—typically asking someone ELSE to do the measuring and documenting. This narrow perspective proves to be a disservice for emotional growth. For reliably accurate measurement of emotional growth, each of us must identify our personal starting point. Only then can we determine how much—if any—we've grown.

> *Ralph and Gwen were a young couple whose relationship started when they were in high school. When their children were born, everything changed. Did he feel like he could handle that huge responsibility? And how was Gwen feeling? As she relied on her family to support her, Gwen began to fully understand who she was and why. But Ralph wasn't sure who HE was! His learning path had lots of bumps, starts and restarts, stops and re-stops. Until he could feel safe in a new comfort zone with a better, deeper understanding of himself, could he fully understand the very big differences between himself and Gwen?*
>
> *So convoluted was Ralph's journey that it took him 25 years of marriage to sort it all out and ask for a divorce. Of course, Gwen's journey was just as complex but very different. Once she realized that they couldn't really be happy or safe together, she agreed to the divorce. Their splitting wasn't contentious or angry, but it was sad.*

Unlike our child-self whose growth was compared to that of other children (a norm-based practice, used mostly to detect and address early-stage health issues), comparative assessment does not serve a useful purpose for emotional growth.

Each adult is as unique as their fingerprints—and it is that uniqueness that drives our individual goals and motivation. For adults, if there is any comparison to be done, it's comparing that which may not be visible but can be expressed like, for example, goals: the gauge is formed by answering for oneself, "What goals have I set and how will I know when I have achieved them?"

THE TALL, TALL TREE
(Is The Tall, Tall Me)

Eunice V. Perez
1930 - 2003

Oh, the tall, tall tree with its stately trunk
And its branches reaching high,
Is a sight to see, tho' the season be
One of four, or day turned night...

The taller the tree the more it can see
And the more it can see is its will
For tho' it must stand in a God-given place,
Its limbs have the whole sky to fill.

The above excerpt is meant to inspire growth—or, better said, it's meant to inspire continuous growth beyond your current circumstances or challenges. The essence of the poem is captured in one short phrase: "...the more it can see is its will..."

So, if life is a journey, how can it also be like a tree that is planted? The two images seem to clash. But when their essential messages are combined, we yield an even more powerful way to measure our personal growth: consider what happens when we align the orientation of the four zones—comfort, fear, learning, and growth—to how we grow as humans.

With the images combined and the orientation adjusted, we can see that growing is an INTENTIONAL EFFORT; it requires us to reach and stretch beyond what's familiar or comfortable—our base/trunk and where we start out. The image also implies that growing is a CHOICE to expand ourselves and our ability. Like a tree, we can measure the number of branches we've created, how far they reach, how effective the shade they cast, and how vibrant the leaves!

This helps us assess our impact. These examples symbolize HOW personal growth is measured—not by how far we've traveled.

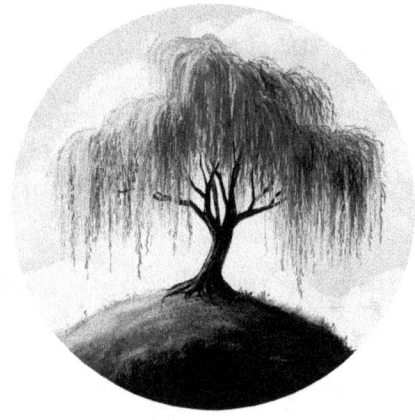

Our ability to form and sustain healthy relationships is largely determined by our own growth. As we discover more and more about our Authentic Self, we always have choices to set new goals that will further our purpose and allow us to live our dreams in a wholesome way.

Complete the following worksheet to begin thinking about and measuring ways you've grown since reaching adulthood.

> ### Anchors - *Takeaways*
>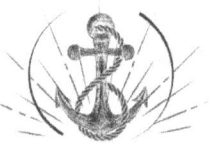
> - GROWTH is a continuous process.
> - RESILIENCE is a growth by-product when a) we acknowledge that negative experiences contribute to our growth; and b) we consider those experiences as lessons. NOTE: The next charter will explore resiliency in depth.

Excursion 15 - My Growth and Progress

Reflection Instructions and Example:

1. Think back over your life's journey thus far. Identify some of the major events that helped you identify your Authentic Self. Maybe it was a difficult divorce your older sister experienced, or it was making a team after two previous rejections.

_____

_____

_____

_____

2. What did those events teach you about yourself? When we look back on our childhood events as an adult, we often get new perspectives and gain insights into who we really are.

_____

_____

_____

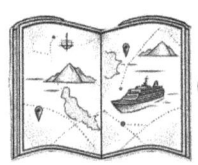 **Charter -RESILIENCE:** *Willows, Palms, and Scrub Oaks*

People that emigrated to new lands for a better life (think: Mayflower, Irish Potato Famine, migrant farm workers, Asian laborers who laid railroads, etc.), all faced seemingly insurmountable odds. In most cases, they arrived needing a sustainable means to survive and gain a foothold. From there, they worked to provide for their needs and wants over their lifetime. Even now and through no fault of their own, they are relegated to the back of an extremely long line during which they must learn a new language and how to overcome obstacles to acceptance and inclusion.

During their journey and throughout their lives, immigrants exhibit a common attribute: resilience. Like immigrants who leave the familiar to establish roots in a hopeful but unknown future, countless lessons are available to us if we recognize the power in our elasticity. No matter whether we are relationship "tumbleweeds" (on the move, searching) or part of a "grove" (planted, committed), we can survive and thrive in the face of challenges and setbacks if we use three specific trees as a reminder: willows, palms, and scrub oaks.

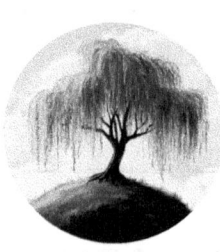 **Willows** have long branches that move and sway in the breeze. When a breeze becomes wind, the branches don't resist it but rather go with the flow of the wind. During our most difficult challenges—those strong winds that threaten to defeat our spirits—we tap into our own elasticity by being aware of the wind but not resistant to it. When the challenges/winds are less intense, we can use that experience as proof of personal strength and stamina: a potential source of pride and self-worth.

Palms are even MORE elastic—not only do their long branches sway with the winds, but their entire body can bend! In fact, even some hurricanes fail to destroy palm trees. When we emerge from emotional Category 5 hurricanes—those episodes that pound us with grief and pain—the experience can leave us forever changed. This is sometimes for the better.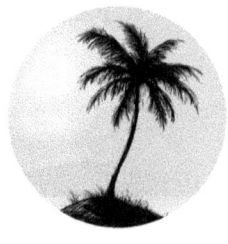

We're better aware of our capabilities under duress. We're better informed to support others. And we're better prepared for similar challenges, all if we can recognize and acknowledge the episode as a strength-test of our elasticity: our resilience.

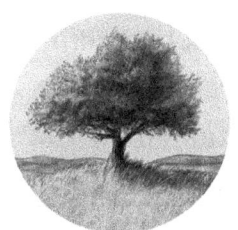

Lastly there are **Oaks—Scrub oaks**. Interestingly, Live oaks, though majestic and strong, have very little bend and can suffer branch damage or topple in high wind. If emotional journeys are the storms of our lives, being a Live oak in a high wind could topple us. This is why we want to tap into our internal Scrub oak. As a Scrub oak, our elasticity is not as obvious as it is when we are Palms. Yet it's there and fortified by tenure—how long we've been working, living, rebounding. A Scrub oak that has continuously weathered lighter storms develops a widely spread network of roots that keep it planted. Over time and despite many hurricanes, Scrub oaks thrive and can be a refuge for others who are ill-prepared for high winds.

That's resilience at work—our elasticity. Each storm we endure makes us better prepared for the next.

Anchors - *Takeaways*

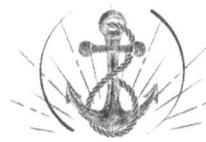

- When we are resilient, we are tapping a power inside of us.
- Challenges and difficulties build resiliency.

Excursion 16 - My Resiliency

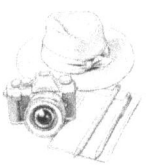

Part of life is facing and overcoming challenges, both the ones we face alone AND the ones we face when we are members of a relationship. Take some time—in fact, make it A PRACTICE—to conduct an inventory of the challenges you've met and overcome. Below is space for you to start creating that habit.

Instructions: In the table below, capture at least three episodes of rough weather: one for which you demonstrated willow resilience, one for palm resilience, and one for Scrub oak resilience. For every demonstration of resilience, push yourself to identify the lesson(s) learned, its contribution to your growth, and the strength that was revealed by that challenge.

Though this table is only a starting point, use it to establish a practice/habit of mentally stepping back from the challenges you have overcome. When you can consistently practice this, you'll know that you've established the root system, base, and branches to weather even the strongest headwinds.

Describe Challenge	What LESSON(s) did you learn?	In what way(s) did the lesson help you GROW?	What STRENGTH(s) were demonstrated or revealed?

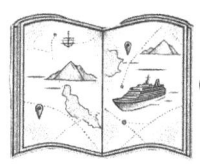 **Charter** - <u>S</u>urviving, <u>L</u>iving, <u>G</u>rowing and <u>T</u>hriving

Do you sometimes feel like you are just getting by? Do you have days when you wake up energized by a purpose, or do you dread facing your daily responsibilities? Our bodies are not designed to be in survival mode for long periods of time. We all have a built-in threat response that can respond to imminent danger. However, some of us may find ourselves living in perpetual survival mode for months (and sometimes years).

When survival mode fully occupies our brain, it robs us of hope. Our survival mode creates the singular goal of getting through another day rather than maximizing our opportunities.

While thriving doesn't exempt us from trouble or stress, it does allow us to navigate through life's challenges. The popular saying "Keep your eyes on the prize" suggests that we need a target—some type of focus for our living rather than merely surviving. LIVING allows us the opportunity to use our resources to meet our needs and to establish healthy connections with others. Living fosters peace of mind, a feeling of being safe and capable of managing our daily responsibilities.

The good news about living is that there is much more to it than feeling safe and capable. Living means we have the capacity to imagine, grow, and exceed our expectations. The human mind is powerful and creative; it's able to render what seems impossible possible. An example of this was when President John F. Kennedy predicted that the United States would send people to the moon: it was a bold and fearless prediction, and we made it happen.

Growing requires us to see beyond what other people see. If we can see it, we can believe it. An individual's vision is based on what they feel capable of ultimately achieving, not on their current status or capability. So let's all ask ourselves:
- Do I have a stretch goal?
- Are my dreams bold?
- Do I allow the doubts of others to limit me?

Growing is a continuous and productive process. Believe it or not, we can grow even while simultaneously experiencing adversity, if we are getting closer to our goal(s). As a matter of fact, problems and challenges can exponentially move us closer. Here's the key: when facing a challenge, instead of focusing on the problem, determine what can be learned from the experience. Growing doesn't only provide an opportunity to learn and share resources/experiences with others—it's a pathway for thriving.

What does it mean to thrive?

Thriving is a mindset of abundance and suggests that one who is thriving is positioned to provide something for others. In healthy relationships, thriving means enhancing each other's lives. Thriving allows us to pour into the other while receiving from them as well. The hallmark of a thriving relationship is that both partners grow individually while giving their best to one another.

Thriving doesn't deplete but rather enhances our life. A thriving couple is like the relationship between the car's battery and alternator: the battery allows the engine to start, and the alternator allows a gas engine to continuously power the vehicle. They work together, like a team, using what each provides to stay in motion!

Note: it is possible to thrive as an individual, and it's not necessary to be in a relationship to feel as though we're thriving. Though we are each responsible for identifying our own life's purpose and leveraging our skills to achieve it, if we ARE in an intimate partnership, our partner should be giving encouragement and support to maintain the relationship's health. Healthy relationships bring out the best in us.

Anchors - *Takeaways*

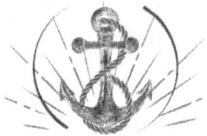

- It's critical to know the difference between living and surviving.
- Growth is based on our INDIVIDUAL vision.
- Thriving in relationships means both people are getting the encouragement and support they need from one another.
- We are made for much more than surviving—we are meant to THRIVE.

Excursion 17 - Surviving, Living Growing, and Thriving (SLGT)

Instructions: For this activity you will rate each of your conditions (Surviving, Living, Growing, and Thriving) on a 10-point scale. One is the lowest, and 10 is the highest. NOTE: THIS IS JUST A "SNAPSHOT" OF WHERE YOU ARE RIGHT NOW. Your conditions may change over time as your life conditions change.

First rate yourself, then describe what you believe is required (from you) to bridge the gap between your actual rating and what you'd rather your condition was. For example, let's look at each of these conditions as if someone is rating themselves:

"SURVIVING" – Suppose my rating = 6.

MY PLAN: For my survival rating to be LOWER (I don't want it to be high), I can be more intentional about increasing my social events. I can push myself to get out and meet more people at least once per week.

"LIVING" – Suppose my rating = 4.

MY PLAN: For my living rating to be HIGHER (I don't want it to be low), I plan to increase my volunteering at the rec center to one weekend per month. Most people who frequent during the day can use a life coach and I can lend that capability.

"GROWING" – My rating = 6.

MY PLAN: For my growing rate to be even HIGHER (I want it to be at least an 8!), I plan to learn a new language. I've heard several people speaking, and I'd really like to understand the language so I can further appreciate the incredible Pinoy vocalists.

"THRIVING" – My rating = 7.

MY PLAN: For my thriving rate to be even HIGHER (I want it to be a 10!), I plan to market my coaching skills. A healthier bank account and more retirement monies will help eliminate some of the practical issues that deplete my energy.

Surviving

1 Low   *5 Moderate*   *10 High*

_____

1st – Rate your current level of **surviving.** 2nd – Describe what you believe is required of yourself to bridge the gap between your current rating and your DESIRED rating. [NOTE: A high Surviving rating is unhealthy for anyone. What must you do for yourself to give it a lower rating in the future?

My plan for A LOWER Surviving rating is _____

_____

Living

1 Low   *5 Moderate*   *10 High*

_____

1st – Rate your current level of **living.** 2nd – Describe what you believe is required of yourself to bridge the gap between your current rating and your DESIRED rating. [NOTE: A low Living rating is unhealthy for anyone. What must you do for yourself to give it a higher rating in the future?

My plan for A Higher Living rating is _____

_____

Growing

1 Low   *5 Moderate*   *10 High*

_____

1st- Rate your current level of **growing.** 2nd – Describe what you believe is required of yourself to bridge the gap between your current rating and your DESIRED rating. [NOTE: A low Thriving rating is unhealthy for anyone. What must you do for yourself to give it a higher rating in the future?

My plan for A Higher growing rating is _____

_____

Thriving

1 Low   *5 Moderate*   *10 High*

_____

1st- Rate your current level of **thriving**. 2nd – Describe what you believe is required of yourself to bridge the gap between your current rating and your DESIRED rating. [NOTE: A low Thriving rating is unhealthy for anyone. What must you do for yourself to give it a higher rating in the future?

My plan for A Higher thriving rating is _____

_____

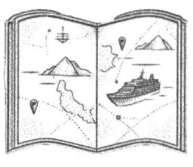 **Charter -** *Life Revelations Activity*

Life Events

List below two or more life events that you think have contributed to your knowledge of who you really are. Perhaps it was the nasty divorce of your parents or another family member, or maybe the loss of someone close to you, or that successful event that you planned and delivered. In any case, the goal here is to not run away from these memories, but to run toward them to see what you can learn about yourself.

Life Revelations

As you review each of these events, find one or two truths that you now realize have contributed to who you really are. Did you comfort the people during that nasty divorce or allow yourself the time to grieve when you lost that loved one, or bask in the applause for your planned event? List below some of those revelations:

___

___

___

Authentic Self:

While revelations provide insights about what we have learned, Authentic Self represents how that experience is an aspect of how we actually show up as an individual. Since the whole idea of this excursion is to connect the dots that represent important learning opportunities, what dots can you connect? Remember that exploring these events courageously may not be easy, but it is very valuable. Many who do this activity only focus on negative events, but positive events are important dots as well.

___

___

___

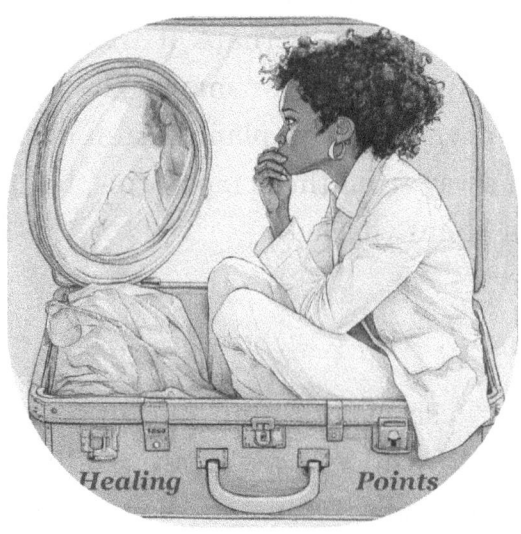

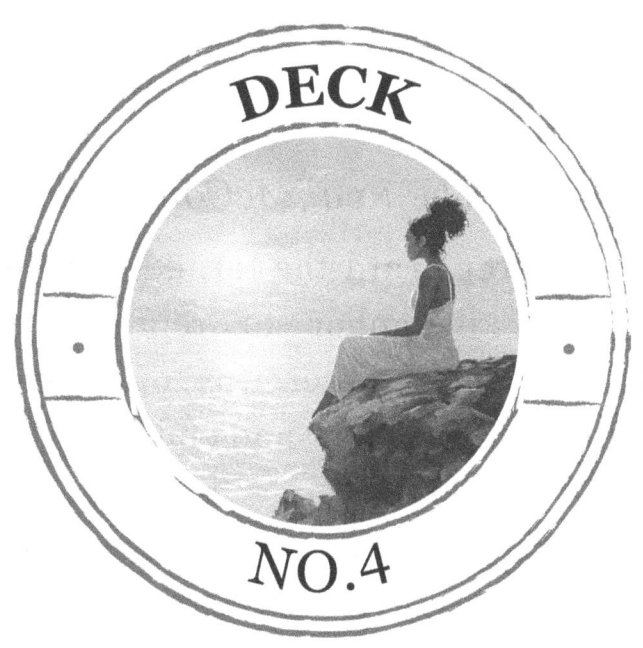

DECK 4

AUTHENTIC SELF DECK

"Vulnerability is the only AUTHENTIC state. Being vulnerable means being open for wounding, but also for pleasure. Being open to the wounds of life means also being open to the bounty and beauty. Don't mask or deny your vulnerability: it is your greatest asset. Be vulnerable: quake and shake in your boots with it. The new goodness that is coming to you in the form of people, situations, and things can only come to you when you are vulnerable, i.e., open."

~ *Stephen Russell, Actor, Writer*

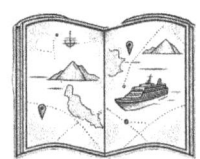 **Charter -** *"The Real McCoy" What is Authenticity?*

Have you ever heard the term, "The Real McCoy," often used as a metaphor to represent the real thing? Authenticity is another way of saying the real thing, meaning that you know and embrace who you are.

The more you know about your true self, the easier it becomes to make life decisions or to evaluate the ones you've already made. Let's look at some of the aspects of personal authenticity:

- You know what you stand for. You will not be pushed into behaviors that violate your standards.
- Your values are yours and yours alone. You have not established them to please others, but to please yourself. As such, you have no need to convince others to adopt your values.
- Your authenticity is your compass and road map. It keeps you on your pathway.
- Your authenticity is the key to healthy, rewarding relationships. Your relationship partner will know who you are and embrace your honesty, even when it doesn't match theirs.
- Once you are rock-solid on who you are and what you stand for, you can expect challenges to your values, often from those closest to you like family and life-long friends.
- Those around you may not understand why you do what you do or say what you say. You may have to practice how to explain/express your authenticity in a straightforward way without judgement.

How to Tell if You are Being Authentic

Authenticity shows up in a relationship when you own who you are and share yourself with a partner without the pressure of retrofitting your standards to your partner's expectations. Authenticity has many benefits but may come with a price when you refuse to fit or stay in a box that others have created for you.

One benefit of authenticity is that you are consistent, and what people see is what they get all day, every day. Authenticity guides you in making the best decisions for you. It protects you from trying to save others at the expense of your health and well-being. Authenticity helps you to establish and maintain boundaries in your relationships. You can clearly see what is yours, and what is someone else's baggage. Authenticity recognizes that you don't have the power to save anyone, but you do have the capacity to be the best version of yourself.

CHALLENGES AND CHOICES OF AUTHENTICITY

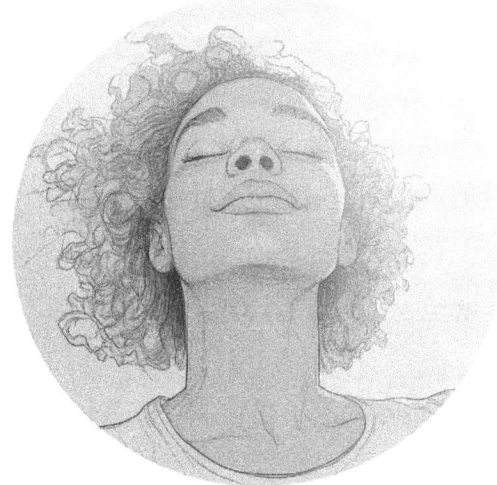

There are some challenges in embracing your Authentic Self. For one, most people will not see or understand you. They will try to define who you are and what they expect you to do.

At times, you may find yourself pushing back against stereotypes and biases. Your peer group may demand compliance with their rules, working hard to maintain homogeneity among its members. These groups can be broad like gender or specific like clubs and associations. If you don't fit the mold, then the assumption is that you are wrong and need to change.

Striving towards Healthy Me includes finding and accepting your Authentic Self, even if other people in your life don't understand or agree. As we embark upon this journey of demonstrating to the world who you are, there may be barnacles, rust, trauma, triggers, and traps to work through. Don't be discouraged if it's taking longer than expected to identify your core values or learn to communicate your feelings or position. Many of us have been wearing a mask for years, and it may take time to learn what's behind the mask. However, once you discover your Authentic Self, your ship will be more fulfilling and productive.

Anchors - *Takeaways*

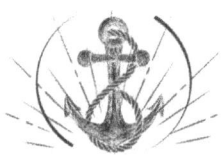

- Establish standards that are uniquely your own.
- Share yourself without pressure or retrofitting your standards to meet others' expectations.

Excursion 18 - Loving Myself

Instructions:

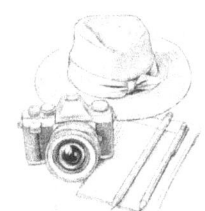

Search the internet or YouTube for the song "Love Myself" by Andy Grammer. Listen to the lyrics and think about how the song reflects your current situation (or not). In what ways do the lyrics resonate with you? What aspect of the lyrics help to articulate what you are experiencing? Capture your thoughts below:

_____

_____

_____

_____

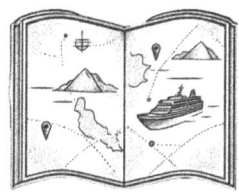

Charter - *Why? The Ralph & Gwen Story*

Every day we make decisions, both big and small, without taking the time to ask ourselves an important question: Why? Too often we act and think automatically, but our thoughts and behaviors stem from multiple sources, including past experiences, lessons learned, our culture, and the values we've developed.

To gain a deeper understanding of how our past influences our present, let's revisit Ralph and Gwen:

> *Ralph was only 16 years old, but he was totally in love with Gwen. He didn't really know how to pursue her and win her love. All he understood was his powerful desire to be with Gwen—that and his hope that she would be equally committed to him.*

Because he's only 16, Ralph is like most young people—not in the habit of questioning his motives or decisions. He hasn't yet learned the value of thinking through the many impact-scenarios embedded in his decisions. He is an example of being not-quite-as-mature as his drive and attraction. This immaturity is often what compels us to make decisions based on what feels good.

Because there are neither reset buttons nor do-overs for our lives, learning to question ourselves is a definite sign of maturity. It allows us to gather more information before determining how to proceed. Even as a teen, learning to ask ourselves "Why?" can set us on a solid path for clearly understanding our values, the motives that underlie our behaviors, and our Authentic Self. If you're like Ralph at age 16—having not yet learned to ask yourself "Why?"—it's not too late to begin doing so. Let's learn more about Ralph and Gwen to see just how powerful the influences on our Authentic Self can impact us if we avoid asking "Why?"

> *Gwen was from a large family who wielded a strong influence on her. Since Ralph only saw Gwen in school or at school activities, he was unaware of the importance of her family to Gwen. In fact, when he stopped to think, 16-year-old Ralph realized that he knew very little about who Gwen really was—but in his mind she was the perfect partner for him. Ralph decided to ask Gwen out, and she said yes.*
> *Before long, Ralph and Gwen were going steady. Everyone loved them together. But Ralph wasn't really interested in public appearances: he was "itching" and only Gwen could satisfy his need to be "scratched." Because Ralph had heard many stories about his parents' torrid, pre-marriage romance, to Ralph, this seemed like a realistic goal for his relationship with Gwen.*

An additional and important piece of information about Ralph and Gwen was their different personalities. Ralph and Gwen were at opposite ends of a spectrum regarding willingness and need to challenge their own adherence to family values.

Ralph was at the end of the spectrum which asks "Why does it have to be this way?" while Gwen was at the other end of the spectrum; she didn't question anything related to family. If Gwen were to be questioned about her behaviors, values, and decisions, she'd have a ready answer: they stemmed from the values and beliefs of her family. So, Gwen represents the folks who don't question teachings and traditions; they adopt them, without consideration that there may be other issues or forces to weigh.

For Consideration

- There's a link between choices and experiences.
- Early experiences drive how we internalize what's right for us.
- Cultural beliefs have molded us.
- Our brains are drawn to what is FAMILIAR—we seek experiences that reflect what (we think) we know.
- Many of us connect with partners that resemble our primary caregiver, despite having sworn to never marry a man/woman like dad/mom.

Let's jump ahead several years in the lives of Ralph and Gwen:

Gwen eventually yielded to Ralph, and they became intimate partners. Just about the time she turned 18 years old, Gwen became pregnant. Ralph was delighted. He wanted nothing more than to be a husband and father. Both families met and concurred that Ralph and Gwen were to marry and had everyone's blessings.

Gwen and Ralph's marriage lasted 25 years. For the first 18 years, they appeared to be a healthy family unit with two kids and good jobs. Both were well-respected in the community. Yet neither Ralph nor Gwen really knew one another—the core of one another.

They had been living to fulfill others' views of a successful marriage. Once they both realized those views were largely a delusion/fairytale, their guilt compelled them to stay together despite their own unhappiness. Gwen began to arrange intimate partnerships with other men while Ralph withdrew into himself and became much less available as a husband or father. Gwen's affairs deeply hurt Ralph, but he never let her or anyone else know.

During those years of self-searching, Ralph began to recognize a pattern of Gwen choosing her family over him. Her behavior wasn't malicious, but it was nonetheless happening. That revelation made Ralph feel deep guilt for not having recognized it much earlier in his marriage. With the revelation came the conviction that he could no longer tolerate a second-class status within his marriage. Ralph filed for divorce after 25 years of marriage to Gwen.

As Ralph and Gwen grew older, they became more capable of seeing both their own Authentic Self and each other's. Though neither of their systems were wrong—Ralph's independence and Gwen's desire to remain close to her family—they were incompatible, a fact they may have realized sooner if they'd taken the time to understand themselves and each other.

Anchors - Takeaways

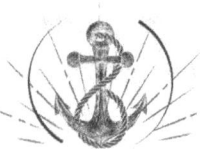

- Our thoughts and behaviors stem from past experiences, lessons learned, our culture, and the values we've developed.
- Early experiences drive how we internalize what's right for us.
- To break unhealthy cycles, it's important to ask ourselves "Why?" Through this process we can find the links between our decisions, experiences, and values.

Excursion 19- *Lessons from Ralph and Gwen*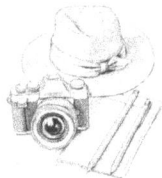

Many of us are living a similar scenario as Ralph and Gwen: we've adopted other people's values, priorities, expectations, and commitments for our lives, all without asking ourselves, "Why?" The years fly by, and we may find ourselves in our middle-ages when we finally decide, like Ralph, to take a hard look and ask questions we've avoided. When is the last time you looked deeply within yourself to ask questions like:

- What's driving my decisions?
- Why do I choose men/women who are struggling with addiction?
- Why am I afraid to apply for a promotion?

Embedded in your answers to the "Why?" are the breakthroughs that will allow you to move forward in your life. "Why?" can be frightening but liberating. Once Ralph got the courage to stop and examine his life, then ask himself how he was feeling about his status in his family, it brought revelations to him that ultimately freed him from guilt, emotional pain, and suffering.

How To Start:

The next time you find yourself battling over a decision you made, ask yourself "Why?" It may sound something like this: "Why was that decision so hard for me to make?" When you give yourself an honest response, ask "Why?" again. Continue asking "Why?" of each response you give yourself—sort of like peeling the onion earlier in this book.

It might sound something like this:

1st Pass:

Q – Why was that decision so hard for me to make?

A – I hate it when I take the wrong actions/make mistakes!

2nd Pass:

Q – Why do you feel so strongly about taking wrong actions or making mistakes?

A – It reminds me of how crazy people around me react. Like when I was a kid and had to do math problems in the front of the room. I never liked it when I needed extra help from the teacher and the other kids didn't.

3rd Pass:

Q – Why didn't you like needing extra help?

A – Kids can be cruel, and they were certainly cruel to me for holding up the class!

4th Pass:

Q – Why do you hang on to that treatment from others?

A – I guess I'm still worried about rejection.

5th Pass:

Q – Why is the rejection fear so strong now?

A – I'm afraid to be alone as I grow older.

Keep going until you've removed the barriers to your truth—the belief/value that is at your CORE.

You'll find a belief or value that was shaped through your life experiences, and it is driving your decisions today. Don't stop asking "Why?" until you reach your truth, your core.

_____
_____
_____
_____
_____
_____

Final Thoughts

At birth we begin the process of forming the core self that will drive our preferences and decisions. Over time we develop values. The old debate between nature and nurture suggests that who we become is a combination of both our DNA and our environment. Sometimes there are environmental elements that we adopt as part of our DNA. We may adopt these elements, but they are NOT in our DNA. Such adoptions can create unhealthy cycles like the relationship in which Ralph and Gwen found themselves.

To break unhealthy cycles, it's important to ask ourselves "Why?" Through this process we can find the links between our decisions, experiences, and values. The goal is not to change our values but to understand what's driving our decisions. "Why?" can also reveal the good, bad, and ugly in our lives. "Why?" can reveal unresolved trauma that has been buried and/or camouflaged by a well-crafted story repeated for years.

That's often how families handle traumatic events: they create a story about it, make sure everyone knows the story, and can repeat it. (See, for example, "We Don't Talk About Bruno" from Disney's Encanto.)

Trauma doesn't dissolve just because it gets buried at sea or locked in our ship's hold. It stays with us. It gets more solidified, like a heavy metal, until we are willing to unpack it. Using "Why?" can get us started.

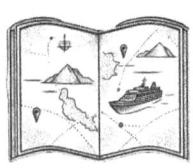 **Charter** - *Getting to the Core*

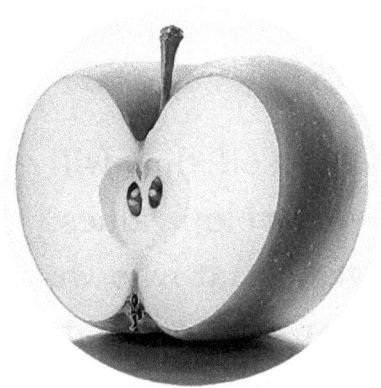 Think about the many ways you've heard the word "core" used. There's the literal, like the core of an apple. When talking about an apple that has spoiled, we might say that it's "rotten to its core." That's because fruits have a center that houses the seeds and a fleshy part that protects the seeds.

Once an apple ripens, if it's not picked and eaten, it will begin to decompose so its seeds can sink into the ground to sprout another version of itself. That's just ONE example of a core and how critical it is to the life cycle of apples—the core holds the seeds of the future.

When we talk about the core of a person, we're really speaking about their essence, which, like the core of an apple, holds the information that can determine their future.

If we're talking about a person's physical core, we're referring to the muscles surrounding the rib cage, which include the diaphragm and pelvic floor. These muscles provide stability and balance for movements like rising from a seated position and the mobility needed to swing a baseball bat. Believe it or not, our core muscles also enable us to perform essential functions like breathing, bowel control, bladder control, and holding our posture.

When we refer to a person's *inner core*, we're referring to the intuition/inner voice that we all have but often ignore. That inner voice is the sound that our personal values make. Although there are values common to most human beings, each of us has a special combination of values that allow us to form an individual personality. Research shows that there is a link between values and personality traits. When we compare personalities, we're really comparing the ways people express their values or inner core. Our core values are essential to maintaining a Healthy Me. Values are important because they drive our actions like how we spend our time and resources.

Our values are shaped by our experiences and who and what we admire; they strongly influence with whom we spend our time. Our values can be reshaped, but they are typically consistent throughout our lifetime. They point us toward what is right and wrong, and they serve as an anchor to our soul. Whether or not anyone else is watching, our values are guiding us.

How do our values play a role in our Authentic Self? Because values are such critical components to what makes up an individual, they play an important role in relationship satisfaction.

For a healthy, satisfying relationship, it's paramount that each person can exercise their values and not be manipulated to violate their core values. For this reason, it is very important that there is alignment between partner values. The more alignment that exists between partners' values, the more intimacy and longevity in the relationship.

Consider this: just like the seeds of an apple, each of our experiences has the potential to produce something that contributes to our future. Whether it be a lesson about ourselves or insights about others, these experiences can produce something that aids in our GROWTH. To identify what's at our core, we must ask ourselves the question, "What matters to me?" Doing so brings us closer to being able to express it with others.

Here's an example that highlights the point:

> *I know a man who, as a child, had a wonderful warm relationship with his Uncle Gus. Uncle Gus and Aunt Ethel came to dinner every Saturday and, as a boy, the man always eagerly anticipated seeing his hero, Gus.*
>
> *But this time was different because Uncle Gus came alone. Ethel was ill in the hospital. As he came into the house, Gus looked so forlorn that the boy was afraid to approach him. He didn't understand all that was happening, but he could only see that his uncle was hurting.*
>
> *Things got worse for Ethel, and when someone asked about her, Gus burst into tears. The boy had never seen an adult cry before, and he knew he had to help. He went up to his bedroom and got Ted, his cherished teddy bear. He brought the bear to his uncle and said that whenever he was sad, Ted always made him feel better. Gus was deeply moved by the gesture, pulled himself together a little, and held the bear close to him throughout the evening.*

Reflecting on this childhood incident of helping his uncle, the man realized something about himself: a big portion of his core is "helper," or someone who will do whatever is in his power to support or assist others.

We can all learn from the Gus and the teddy bear story. Lessons about our core are embedded in so many situations we encounter —we need only take the time to examine them

> ### *Anchors* - *Takeaways*
>
>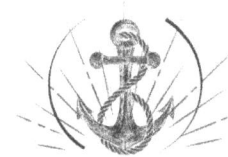
>
> - At our core is our deepest truth.
> - Consistently bringing our truest self in all we do plants the seeds for richer, more satisfying relationships.

Excursion 20 - Getting to The Core - What I Value

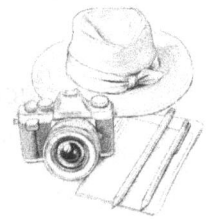

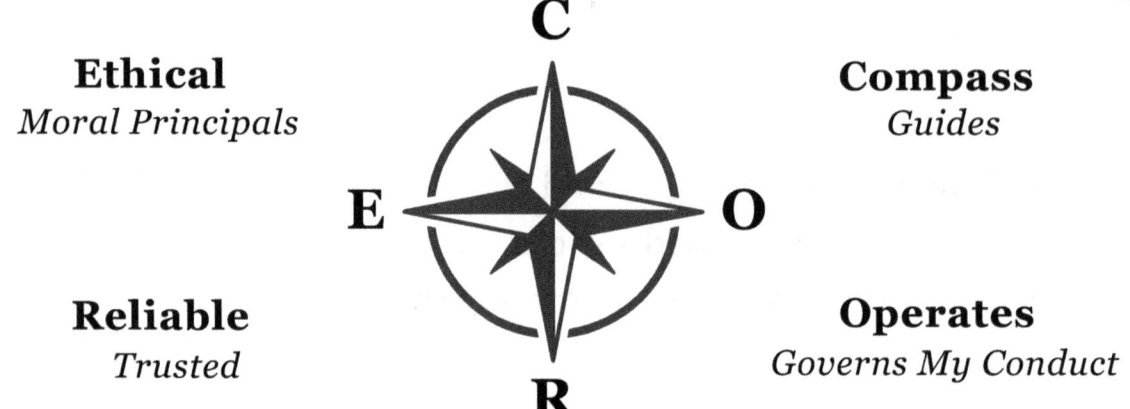

Ethical
Moral Principals

Compass
Guides

Reliable
Trusted

Operates
Governs My Conduct

INSTRUCTIONS:

Recall the mindfulness activities we've done in earlier Charters of this book: take a few minutes to get in touch with YOURSELF. Think about WHAT IS AT YOUR CORE. Capture three to four values and/or attributes that fulfill the description of C.O.R.E. that you can share. These values/attributes are part of your Authentic Self. To help, we've created an acronym that compels you to think of the elements of yourself that comprise your core:

C – Compass	*Helps me stay on a chosen course; no matter what. Used to gauge if something is right/wrong for me.*
O – Operates	*Drives my behavior.*
R – Reliable	*Stays with me on good and bad days*
E – Essence	*Without it, I wouldn't be Me.*

Detailed Example:

"At my core are Integrity, Kindness, Gratefulness, and Humor. They guide my conduct, and I seek those attributes, behaviors/values from others."

How my core shows up in my behaviors and style:

My CORE compelled me as a parent. I raised my children to understand the importance of learning from their mistakes and owning a part of any outcome. Introspection was the focus of discussions/debriefs regarding challenging situations they experienced. I approached the conversation with:

- *What lesson(s) did you learn?*
- *What would you do differently now that you have hindsight?*

The impact of using my CORE as superpower has been:

- *Mutually open, honest, and supportive relationships with my adult-aged children*
- *A circle of trusted friends on whom I can rely during good times and difficulties*

What values are at your CORE?

_____

_____

How has your core shown up in your behaviors and values?

_____

_____

The impact of using my CORE as superpower has been:

_____

_____

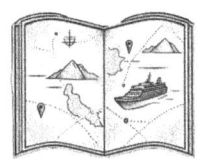 **Charter** - *Nourishing My Authentic Self*

The phrase "the seat of government" doesn't refer to an actual chair, but rather to the center of what happens—where the rules are made. Like the government, people also have a personal seat of government that contains the rules by which we conduct ourselves and our lives; it's called our SOUL. At the center of all humans, there is an invisible force that helps us know when something is either aligned or in conflict with us as individuals.

People also have a non-verbal way of demonstrating what's at our seat of government/soul: it's called SPIRIT. Spirit is an outward manifestation or energy of what's inside our soul. There are folks whose spirit seems to mesh very well with those around them, and there are those whose spirit may not. If you've ever met someone with whom you just "click," you've experienced the phenomenon of having kindred spirits.

In situations like this, we have no outward evidence to support our feelings—this is our intuition. Our intuition often operates as direct communication to us, much like an alarm or caution light that indicates we should focus and pay closer attention. Many people whose intuition is activated will express that a situation or person just didn't sit right with them. Knowing how the spirit is tethered to the seat of our personal, individual rules regarding what's right or wrong, such a statement really means: What's happening doesn't feel aligned with who I am. What we're describing here is our Authentic Self. It sounds simple, but being clear about our Authentic Self can be challenging because most people have been inundated with the expectations of family, society, affiliations, and the like.

In fact, many of the tangible rewards we receive in life result from behaving how the world expects us to, such as good grades in school and promotions at work. What's more, many of us fail to heed our inner voices (soul/spirit connection) and instead create fake personalities that are rooted in the expectations of others and shaped by what's easiest or will generate the least challenge by others.

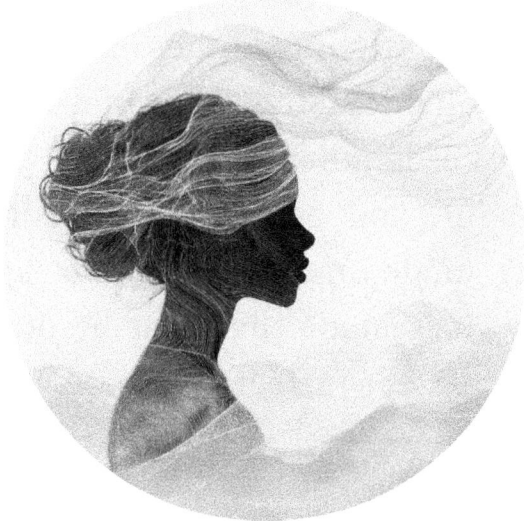

As time passes, we use these superficial personalities so much that they may compel us to make decisions that are totally opposite of what would better satisfy or nourish our soul.

Why is the soul so important to Authentic Self? To answer that, let's think about children. They genuinely express their emotions without filters. Most children experience life in the moment, with abandon and without fretting about what the next experience will bring. Until children encounter society's choke-hold of norms and expectations, they view life through the lens of their authentic perspective.

Because our soul is the seat of ourselves, we use it (many times, unconsciously) to help make decisions that align with what's at our core: our values. As such, our soul is like the architect of our personality. Our soul helps us establish the meaning and purpose of our lives. Via the spirit we reveal our will, motivation, and determination—all of which has the same source: our soul. Because our soul is the source of the energy we emit via our spirit, it is critical that each of us is clear about what's in our soul, and what nourishes our soul.

Our spirit not only reflects what's in our soul, but it is also the invisible force that animates our bodies. Since it's an energy—like electricity—spirit can be depleted. Like fuel for a car, our spirit's depletion can often be demonstrated by our outward demeanor, attitude, comportment, and other physical signs. When we are physically ill, it is made manifest by our spirit. When we're mentally distracted, it is made manifest by our spirit. When our spirit is too depleted, it affects our physical, mental, and emotional well-being.

We can use our spirit to support and ensure the wellness and balance of our soul. Let's use the recent example of the 2020 Olympics when Simone Biles—the overwhelming favorite of the Games—pulled herself out of the team competitions:

Despite the barrage of negative press and banter she received, gymnast Simone Biles demonstrated an acute understanding that if her mind was not focused, she could neither control nor rely upon her body to eliminate potentially fatal errors. Spinning in the air at high speeds and heights without full ability to focus could have resulted in her being maimed or killed.

At a minimum, Biles could not expect the best of herself, so she took a step back to restore her mental focus which would, in turn, allow her to restore control over execution of the correct physical techniques. With control of the physical, Biles realized she could perform her routines with confidence, stick her landings, and celebrate the solid execution of her routines. With each successful execution of her routines, her confidence grew, her focus increased, and her spirits rose. Biles recognized that her mental health was connected to her physical performance, which was, in turn, connected to her emotional wellness. She realized that her erratic performance was due to the following domino effect:

> *--lack of mental focus,*
>
> *--which impacted her performance,*
>
> *--which impacted her confidence,*
>
> *--which impacted her emotions,*
>
> *--which brought down her spirits.*

Tending to just one of the symptoms allowed Biles to restore her balance and win a medal in the individual competition.

Similarly, the UCONN Husky Women's Basketball Head Coach has a purposeful recruiting process:

> *When Head Coach of UCONN Women's Basketball, Geno Auriemma, interviews a possible recruit for the UConn Women's Basketball team, they do not talk about basketball. In fact, the interview happens with the young woman's entire family. Coach Auriemma already knows the prospective team member can play basketball, but the support and understanding she'll need to be successful in his program is more about the recruit's awareness of her Authentic Self and her family's desire to support that awareness. He wants to understand the recruit's spirit, because that's the key to her success.*

So how can you tell if your lifestyle and your soul are out of sync? You'll often experience feelings like insecurity, bitterness, restlessness, lack of intimacy, isolation, and a hyper-critical attitude. On the other hand, how can you tell if your soul is nourished and satisfied? You'll exude emotions like joy, compassion, peace, purpose, fun, and connection with others; you'll have energy to engage in activities, generosity towards others, and a clear vision for how to pursue what is important in your life.

It is critically important to NOURISH your soul so it can serve as your guide. To nourish and sustain the soul you must:

- Have a clear purpose
- Introspect/Self-Reflect
- Meditate
- Rest
- Have gratitude
- Have time to yourself
- Have honest, in-depth communication

How might you be able to tell that your pursuits are nourishing your soul? When you engage in the pursuits, are you compelled to say/think:

- "I felt it in my spirit."
- "My spirit was lifted."

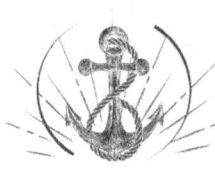

Anchors - *Takeaways*

- Because our soul is the source of the energy we emit via our spirit, it is critical that we are clear about what nourishes our soul.
- Our soul helps us establish the meaning and purpose of our lives.
- Our spirit not only reflects what's in our soul but is also the invisible force that animates our bodies.

Excursion 21 - Reflection

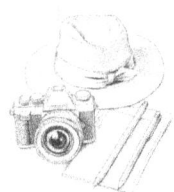

Create a mental list of your activities/pursuits from today. Ask yourself:

1. Did I do things that I wanted to do or had to do?
2. Of the things I did that I had to do, did they align with what is important to ME or to others?
3. When I think about my pursuits, do I feel energized/happy, or weighed down/overwhelmed?
4. Who do I trust/rely on? Why? What about our connection am I most grateful for?
5. What do I do to rest? Why? How can I increase the time I allow for myself?

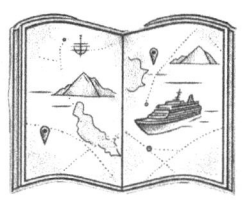

Charter - *Unapologetically Loving My PDP*

"This is Me!"

- *The Greatest Showman, 2017*

My <u>P</u>urpose, <u>D</u>irection, and <u>P</u>assions

P is for PURPOSE

How many times have you let your best friend or a family member talk you out of a project or investment that you believed in? Far too many people are so focused on convincing others to agree with them that their vision never actually becomes reality.

Your purpose is not a group activity. This doesn't mean you can't accept help or feedback as you aspire to be your best, but you shouldn't be dependent on others to define or validate your mission or vision in life. Sometimes, the people closest to you will not understand or even agree with your direction and purpose.

> *Consider Walt Disney before he became internationally known. Most investors did not share his vision about amusement parks for parents and children. They scoffed at his idea. Those naysayers did not deter Disney. Over time, he added to his original ideas and eventually achieved bigger and bolder dreams.*

Remember, your purpose is unique to you and the only person's approval you need is YOURS. OWN IT. PURSUE IT. Others can follow—or not. Even if you want followers and supporters, you must be committed to your vision. People follow when the leader is committed. Think Moses, Harriet Tubman, Sojourner Truth. They all faced obstacles, but they treated their obstacles as opportunities that provided clarity on how best to move around, over, or under. Obstacles were never barriers to achieving their respective purpose.

D is for DIRECTION

Learning about your Authentic Self is an ongoing process that continues throughout life. The person you understood yourself to be at 16 has more facets at 26 and even more facets at 46! As the years move on—and if you are paying attention—your self-awareness should also be increasing. With greater self-awareness, you will find more comfort behaving authentically—based on your truths—rather than following paths or people not aligned with your truths. You'll also find it easier to maintain the direction you choose and with less temptation to veer from what you know to be right for YOU. Self-awareness and being true to oneself both allow us to be happier and consistent as we share ourselves with others. If you're currently hiding behind a mask, take it off! Reveal who you are to the world. You'll likely learn that many others welcome your openness, honesty, and authenticity!

P is for PASSION

Purpose and direction are insufficient if you have no passion for what you do. Yet passion isn't about feeling good due to positive feedback or accomplishments. Passion is what drives us to persevere amid failures and setbacks. It fuels us when it seems we are out of options. Passion doesn't depend on a paycheck but rather it compels us to do it even if there were no payment. Passions speak to the "So what?" in a project.

> *In 1984, Wendy's launched a successful marketing campaign highlighting the famous phrase "Where's The Beef?!" Basically, Wendy's was touting the superiority of its burgers (due to the amount of meat they contained) over its competitors. Wendy's beefier burgers campaign provides an analogy for passion: Anybody can have a clear purpose and commit to a direction—but we must ask, "Where's The Passion?!"*

Passion provides that element which compels others to join you and be a part of your success.

What's the Point of PDP?

Before you make the decision to invest in a relationship with another person, invest time in YOURSELF, learning more about or enhancing your understanding of your Authentic Self. Never apologize for your Authentic Self. Own your purpose. Have direction and passion. All these combined represent Healthy Me.

Anchors - *Takeaways*

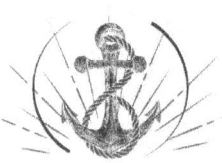

- Purpose: Know why you exist and commit your energy and resources to fulfill your unique mission in life.
- Direction: Have a plan for How to fulfill your purpose.
- Passion drives us to persevere.
- Relationships neither complete you nor fulfill your purpose but rather, give you an opportunity to share your life with someone special as you each fulfill your purposes.

Excursion 22 - Reflection Cont.

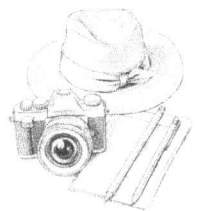

If you're in a relationship and any of the following is consistently occurring, reconsider whether that relationship is a REALationship:

- Your partner spends more time trying to distract you from your purpose rather than supporting you in achieving it.
- You find yourself modifying your goals because your partner feels threatened by your potential or real success.
- You find yourself constantly adapting to what your partner expects of you.

Excursion 23 - Activity: Finding My Purpose

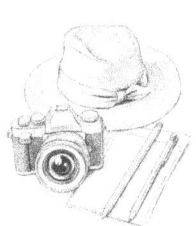

(Adapted from Life Path and Career Purpose Consultants)

The illustration on the following page resembles a blossom and was adapted from a concept about our life's purpose. It is essentially meant to represent the approach we should take to better identify our own unique reason for being, which is reflected by our purpose. To apply the illustration for finding your purpose, you must be able to give serious thought to the four questions represented by the four ovals:

- What are you good at? = Skills you have
- What do you love to do? = Passions you have
- What's something others need or want? = It's in demand

- Can you be compensated for it? = It satisfies your financial needs

As you examine the expanded Venn diagram, you'll notice that the four ovals overlap. For example, if you were to combine a skill (singing) with a passion (performing), that represents a talent (entertaining others). For every overlap, there is a suggestion of how that combination of overlapping ovals might show up in your behaviors. The four ovals overlap at a "sweet spot," which is noteworthy because that pursuit (which combines all of the abovementioned ovals) might just be your reason for being—your purpose.

HOW TO USE THE ILLUSTRATION:

1. Think about two or three time-consuming activities in which you are currently involved.
2. Examine each one of the activities separately, asking yourself which of the four colored ovals your activity represents. NOTE: your activity may represent more than one of the colored ovals.
3. If after considering each of the activities, you have determined that none represent a sweet spot, you have just proven to yourself that where you're spending much of your time is not necessarily your purpose.
4. Continue to examine all of the activities in which you engage until you've exhausted your current pursuits. If NONE seem to satisfy that sweet spot definition, you may want to determine what's needed for you to start pursuing more of that which does satisfy your sweet spot/purpose.

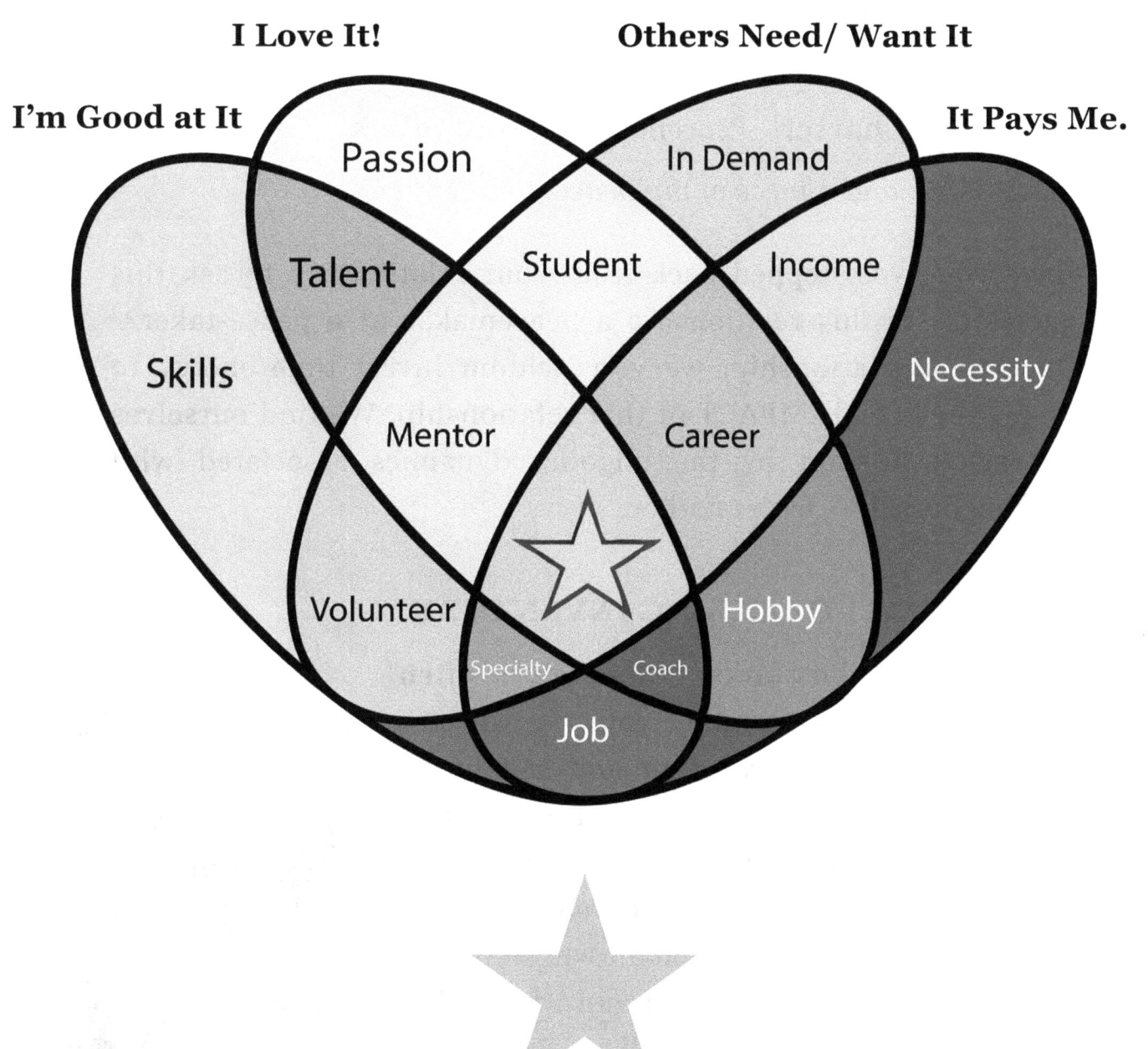

In the next charter, you'll have an opportunity to focus on the pursuit of your purpose and the importance of that pursuit to your peace of mind

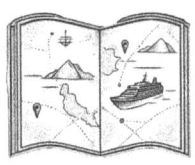 **Charter -** *Peacemakers, Peace-takers,*

and a piece of my peace

Have you ever stepped back from your relationship to ask this question: "Is this relationship a peacemaker or a peace-taker?" Once in a relationship, we very seldom invest time/energy to assess the actual IMPACT of that relationship. We find ourselves distracted or rapt by the ongoing dynamics associated with sharing ourselves with another.

THE BENEFIT OF TAKING INVENTORY

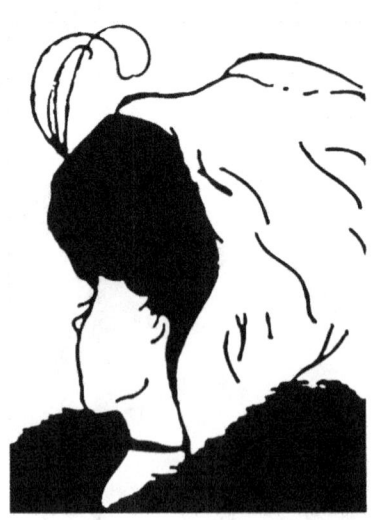

The renowned illustration to the right is often shown to help people gain a deeper understanding of perception and judgment. Many glance at the illustration and immediately see the profile of a young woman. Others fail to see the young woman and, instead, see an old woman whose hair is partially covered with a scarf and whose chin is tucked down into her collar. Even after explaining that both perceptions are true, some people might fail to see two images.

We can all benefit from taking time to step back and review that with which we've become familiar. Like the illustration, our relationships have characteristics that we might overlook or ignore. Taking the time to closely examine specific aspects of the relationship—especially when it has existed for several milestones e.g., together for many years, have children/pets we share, joint ownership of a business/property, etc.—is one of the healthiest exercises we can give our relationships. If we fail to inventory our relationships, we can get stuck seeing the same old things and neglect all the new.

PINPOINT THE NOISE

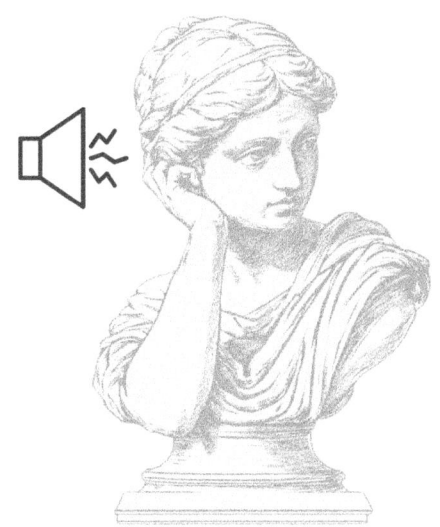

The most basic definition of noise: an unpleasant sound that causes disturbance. There is probably nothing more frustrating than experiencing noise that disturbs your peace. In relationships, peace is represented by those times when expectations are met or exceeded, boundaries are respected, and personal pet peeves are not triggered. The disturbances that represent relationship noise can occur much like spontaneous combustion—we're not certain of the exact cause, but we know that a build-up of something creates the blaze.

Being able to anticipate noise empowers us to address it. The healthiest relationships are the ones that expect noise and welcome the opportunity it provides for gaining insights into the other person's expectations, boundaries, or personal pet peeves. Such an investment yields bountiful returns because it gives everyone an opportunity to work through the challenge or trigger of the noise. Once addressed together, it is easier to anticipate and/or avoid similar mistakes.

THE JOURNEY

REALationships are like co-travelers. The nature of relationships is that they are constantly moving and changing—never really in the same waters because people are constantly moving and changing too. The person with whom you fell in love last year has had an entire year to see, do, and be—emerging with more insights about themselves and, hopefully, YOU. With this reality comes a bit of inconvenience: just when you'd like the other person to stay put, there they go, sailing again!

Acceptance is the key to a good journey. Some relationships are strengthened by rough seas because each person gains experience—and gets proof of the seaworthiness of their vessel, the relationship. Others experience a lack of preparedness. Still others may remain on a doomed journey rather than face the prospect of traveling solo.

These concepts can help as you work through the questions posed in the inventory below. Honesty provides the most value for the time you invest. As you rate your relationship, keep in mind the ultimate goal: clarity about the degree to which your relationship is a peacemaker or peace-taker. Once completed, only you can determine if the relationship is worthy of investing A PIECE OF YOUR PEACE. If it is not, investing your energy in peacemaking self-care may be the best direction to steer your vessel!

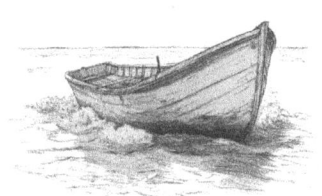

Using your inventory results, determine parts of this book that can help you develop healthier habits to enrich your REALationship, express your needs clearer, or take the necessary steps to administer self-care for holding onto your peace.

Anchors - *Takeaways*

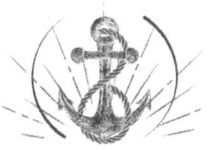

- Taking inventory is one of the healthiest exercises we can give our relationships.
- The healthiest relationships expect and welcome noise as an opportunity for understanding expectations, boundaries, or personal pet peeves.
- Acceptance is the key to a good journey.

Excursion 24 - Rate Your Relationship - Peacemaker or Peace-Taker?

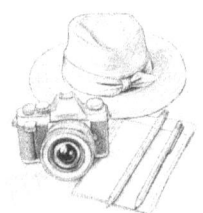

INSTRUCTIONS:

The following activity provides an opportunity for you to begin taking inventory and determine if there are areas that may need your attention. Circle the appropriate number below for each question. Once you've circled a rating for each, you have completed an initial inventory of important aspects of relationships in life. Upon completion, you will also be clearer on those aspects of your life that are peacemakers, and those that are robbing you of your peace.

PEACEMAKER	PEACE-TAKER
Has clarity and purpose 1---------2---------3---------4---------5 low high	Purpose and values are unclear 1---------2---------3---------4---------5 low high
Does what's necessary, even when it's difficult 1---------2---------3---------4---------5 low high	Does what's convenient and personally comfortable 1---------2---------3---------4---------5 low high
Look for ways to bring the relationship to a place of homeostasis—stability 1---------2---------3---------4---------5 low high	Gets stuck in their righteous feelings; unable to resolve conflict, and often create escalation of conflict 1---------2---------3---------4---------5 low high

PEACEMAKER	PEACE-TAKER
Accepts responsibility for own behaviors and points the finger at oneself when assessing blame 1---------2---------3---------4---------5 **low** **high**	Blames everyone except self for situations that go wrong. 1---------2---------3---------4---------5 **low** **high**
Seeks good in others and wants to see them win 1---------2---------3---------4---------5 **low** **high**	Finds difficulty seeing good in others; distrusts motives of others 1---------2---------3---------4---------5 **low** **high**
At peace with self 1---------2---------3---------4---------5 **low** **high**	At odds/in conflict with others and self 1---------2---------3---------4---------5 **low** **high**
Avoids hidden agendas 1---------2---------3---------4---------5 **low** **high**	Pursues personal agenda that may not be productive or comfortable for others 1---------2---------3---------4---------5 **low** **high**
Accepts Authentic Self of partner—warts and all 1---------2---------3---------4---------5 **low** **high**	Tries to mold partner into what he/she wants them to be 1---------2---------3---------4---------5 **low** **high**
Understands boundaries and "staying in their own lane" of life 1---------2---------3---------4---------5 **low** **high**	Noses into others' business as if others should bend to their preferences 1---------2---------3---------4---------5 **low** **high**

PEACEMAKER	PEACE-TAKER
State of mind and a "way-of-lifer" that don't fret over the little things 1---------2---------3---------4---------5 **low** **high**	Frets over things that may have little-to-no priority 1---------2---------3---------4---------5 **low** **high**
Has enough life experiences to know what's important 1---------2---------3---------4---------5 **low** **high**	Despite experience, treats situations as a novice who believes all issues have equal importance 1---------2---------3---------4---------5 **low** **high**
Knows life isn't fair and that we should expect some struggles 1---------2---------3---------4---------5 **low** **high**	Expects life to run smoothly for themselves 1---------2---------3---------4---------5 **low** **high**
Seeks opportunities to be at peace with self and others 1---------2---------3---------4---------5 **low** **high**	Finds a way to create conflict wherever they roam 1---------2---------3---------4---------5 **low** **high**

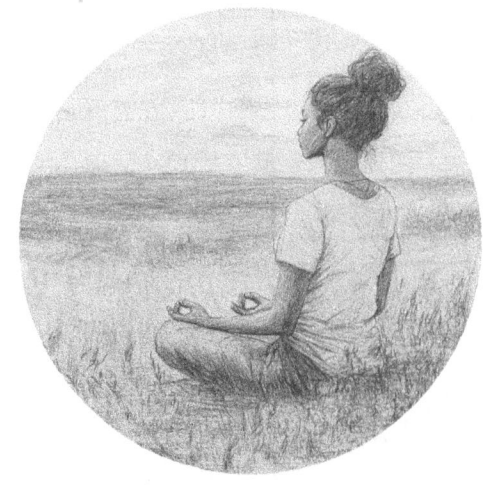

Excursion 25A - My Authentic Self - Statement Development (Healthy Me)

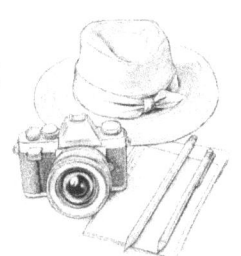

The popular ballad by Whitney Houston entitled, "Try It on My Own" is about overcoming self-doubt and fear to authentically approach life. As mentioned earlier, authenticity is another way of being REAL; knowing and embracing who you are. The better we know our true selves, the easier it is to make life decisions or to evaluate the ones we've already made.

INSTRUCTIONS:

Create a succinct statement below that helps you provide others with a high-level understanding of YOU. Your final statement should reflect as many of the following as possible:

- You know what you stand for and you don't violate those standards.
- Your values are yours and were established by you, for you.
- You live your values to satisfy yourself and not others.
- You clearly recognize when/if you have gotten off your pathway.
- Your authenticity fuels both your health and rewarding relationships.

Authentic Self Statement Outline

Passion: What EXCITES you to get involved/care? *"I am driven by..."*

Sample Response: Trustworthiness and compassion.

Your Response:

_____

_____

Values: What's CRITICAL for you to be able to exercise/apply in your interactions with others? *"I strongly believe..."*

Sample Response: Helping people feel heard.

Your Response:

_____

_____

Growth: What are you committed to doing/being a part of? *"I will..."*

Sample Response: Seek to acknowledge and own my contribution to outcomes that fall short of aspirations. I am worthy of happiness, comfort, and space to pursue my interests.

YOUR RESPONSE:

_____

_____

Self-Declaration: *Who Are You?*

Sample - *"I am driven by trustworthiness and compassion. I strongly believe in helping people feel heard. I seek to acknowledge and own my contribution to outcomes that fall short of aspirations. I am worthy of happiness, comfort, and space to pursue my interests."*

YOUR SELF-DECLARATION:

_____

_____

_____

_____

_____

_____

Healthy We:
IDENTIFYING VESSELS IN YOUR FLEET

Why do so many people struggle to maintain good relationships? The short answer: It's complicated. The good news is that despite the complexity, there are ways to succeed if you bring honesty and a willingness to work on it. What's the "it?" It is the relationship—a combination of YOU and your approach with OTHERS. Healthy We helps you understand, repair, and maintain relationships that are important to you.

Healthy We uses ships for its main analogy to describe four common types of relation investment: friendSHIP, companionSHIP, situationSHIP, and intimate partnerSHIP. As we describe healthy relationships, we term them REALationships because the deliberate misspelling conveys the quest: trust and commitment that is GENUINE, not an act or knockoff.

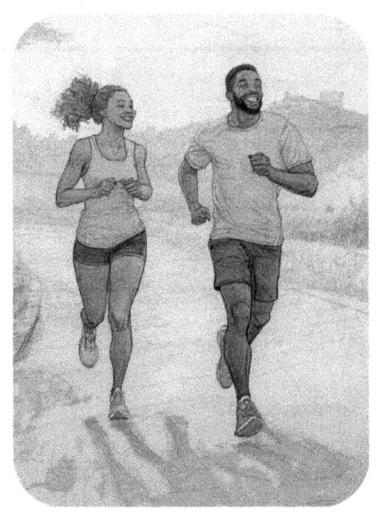

Whether you're just starting the journey toward a friendship/situationship, or developing an existing companionship/intimate partnership, it's crucial that your ultimate vessel be capable of withstanding challenges and adverse conditions. It is for this reason we use the deliberate misspelling "C-worthy" as short-hand for commitment-worthy: worth the effort and cost of maintenance.

So, ask yourself: Are you ready for a REALationship? Is your current relationship C-worthy? If you want to embark on a journey filled with trust and commitment, you should have discovered at least some of your Authentic Self. Applying your understanding, trust, and love of SELF will all be necessary to manage the challenges, conflicts, and choices that naturally occur on the journey toward a friendship, situationship, companionship, and intimate partnership. The decks, charters, and excursions in this part of the book reflect nautical concepts associated with embarking on the high seas. They offer specific advice to help apply your Authentic Self while managing your SHIPS.

If you're ready for a C-worthy REALationship, let's get started. Although you will certainly encounter challenges, each challenge provides an opportunity to choose and refine behaviors that bring you to breathtaking ports. While you may be tempted to undertake lesser challenges, remember that any ship you board will require ongoing maintenance. Hopefully, however, the rewards of ongoing maintenance will be well worth the effort!

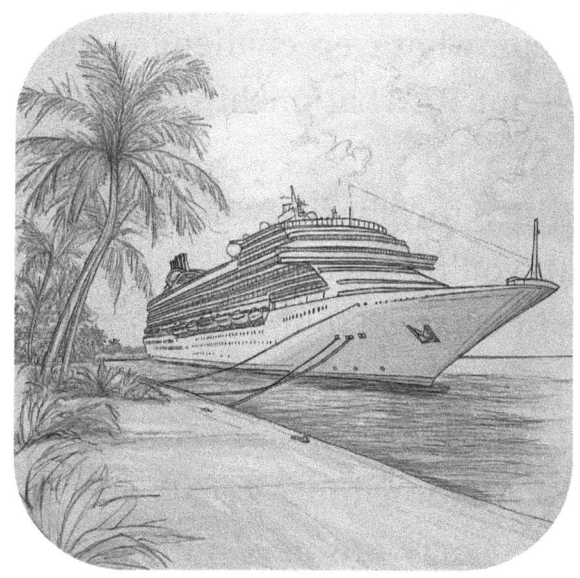

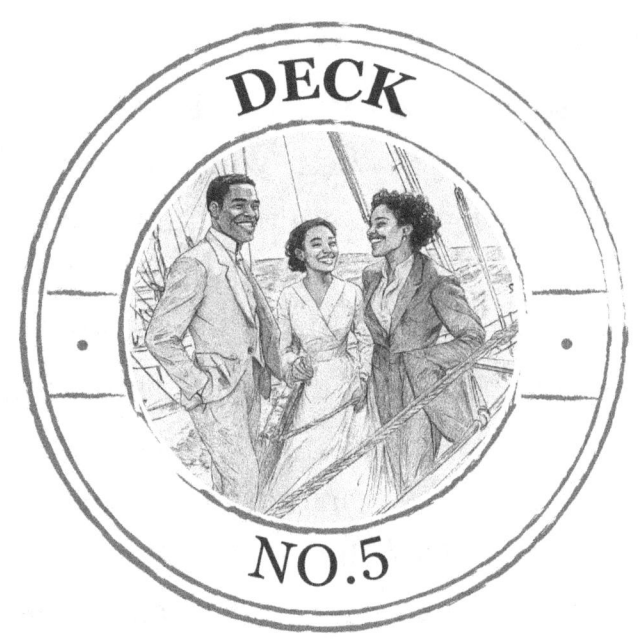

DECK 5

SHARE DECK

SHARE is where friends, couples, companions, etc., begin. When we involve ourselves with others, we share who we are, our values, and vision for our life. This includes our blemishes and warts. Our strengths, lessons learned, and individual needs are all part of the invitation we extend to the trusted others and hope that they will accept whatever challenges they may encounter during the voyage—our REALationship.

There is no substitute for sharing. If you use the excuse of not having time, what you're saying is, "I don't have the time to sustain the GOOD in what we found…"

It is wise to share your barnacles. It represents being vulnerable and it's good for REALationships. Recall that barnacles are flaws that you realize--that may not need immediate attention—but if not addressed can impact the health of the relationship.

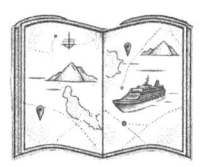 # Charter - *Situationship*

Situationships can Lead to Healthy Choices

Relationships are complex and may seem even more complicated than they were several decades ago. To be fair, relationships were NEVER simple, even in the past; what's changed is our deeper respect for authenticity and the importance of bringing our whole selves into relationships.

There have always been relationships outside of the mainstream, but nowadays alternative relationships have an increasingly greater acceptance rate. For example, it's common to hear someone talk about friends-with-benefits, or situationships, swinging, open relationships, and polyamory. How are such relationships different, and how do these differences contribute to a healthy lifestyle?

Healthy relationships are not defined by the so-called moral majority; rather, they are defined by whether they produce healthy outcomes.

Friends-with-benefits typically involve some type of sexual behavior without emotional commitment or investment, while situationships typically indicate more exclusivity regarding intimacy, but still without commitment or a declared future. Open relationships have committed partners who allow for sexual encounters with others but do not permit commitment beyond sex. Swinging is similar except there is minimum sharing outside of the sexual experience—in short, it's all about having sex with varied partners. Polyamory, on the other hand, centers on establishing multiple, committed, and concurrent relationships. Despite these relationships being considered taboo, data has suggested that one in five adults have been part of a consensual, non-monogamous relationship.

Another component of situationships is that they are romantic, casual exchanges and typically short-term. Similar to an excursion on a cruise ship, situationships serve as a means of having fun without expectations of a future. Such relationships tend to be inconsistent and non-exclusive. situationship participants often have a style of "Don't ask, don't tell." While this may work for some, one or both parties frequently experience confusion and feelings of anxiousness regarding the future of the relationship. While deeper desires may exist, partners may be unclear about what to do with their feelings. Why? One reason is science has proven that separating emotions from physical connections is harder than it sounds!

Recalling "Your Brain in Love" Cruise Document, living beings are designed to connect with others. The biological explanation is that physical intimacy produces endorphins and dopamine in the brain, which generate what we know as feelings for a person. What's more, when we are attracted to someone, the brain creates the hormone oxytocin. Endorphins, dopamine, and oxytocin are all naturally derived from within each of us and cause our desire for a deeper connection. Research shows that the hormones oxytocin and vasopressin heighten sexual arousal and the process of falling in love. Although we may try to keep our interests at a surface level, sex itself is never just physical but rather creates unexpected connections.

So here's the important question: can situationships be healthy relationships? When you think about the components of a healthy relationship (trust, safety, security, and commitment), it may be difficult to recognize how a situationship can produce a long-term, healthy connection. Yet situationships are not always bad. There is much good that can be extracted from a situationship, but those choosing such a vessel must be clear about their purpose and must be realistic about their expected outcomes. What's more, situationships can provide necessary space and time to evaluate just what type of "ship" we desire: a soloship (no ties, no commitments), a friendship, a companionship or partnership.

HOW TO LEVERAGE A SITUATIONSHIP

Recall the mindfulness activities we've done in earlier Charters of this book: take a few minutes to get in touch with YOURSELF. Think about WHAT IS AT YOUR CORE? Also consider these bullets:

- ***A situationship can be like a port of call*** - That's an opportunity to get off the ship and take time to explore and/or evaluate. Such an excursion provides a chance to heal and recalibrate before catching the next ship. While in such a situationship, recognize there may be distractionships like party boats or speed boats. These excursions can complicate your journey!
- **Beware the Party Boat** - Party boats offer temporary fun and avoidance like alcohol or substances to self-medicate. All this serves to do is delay the healing you may be seeking.
- **Beware the Speed Boat** - Similar to playing the renowned board game Monopoly, during which you pull the card that allows you to collect your money and avoid all the risks of landing on properties that require payment of rent (head directly to GO!), the Speed Boat leaves no time/space to assess and heal any emotional wounds. Such a boat leaves you susceptible to making poor decisions and perpetuation of the damaging cycle.

Use a situationship to reflect on your Authentic Self and to determine which type of ship you need to board. There are no right or wrong answers.

Anchors - Takeaways

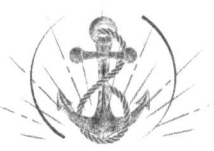

- Non-traditional and non-monogamous relationships are on the rise because they offer flexibility to connect with people on their terms.
- We may move from one ship to another depending on our needs.
- After investing in embracing our Authentic Self and understanding our core, it's time to engage in healthy relationships.

Excursion 25B- Situationships: A Time of Reflection

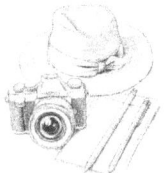

Are you between relationships? Or maybe you're in a relationship that's not working for you. Feeling stuck often stems from feeling obligated to make relationship decisions based on others' expectations. If you answered yes to any of these questions, situationships can be an opportunity to decide what you need right now.

INSTRUCTIONS: This excursion can help you better determine which type ship is best for you. Listed below are different ships we might board. Identify the ship you feel is best for you and explain why you made your choice.

- **Speed Boat** *Situationship* (Making choices in the moment; open to new experiences and want to avoid making any serious decisions).
- **Party Boat** *Friends with Benefits* (Looking for temporary fun; not ready for a serious relationship).
- **Sailboat** *Friendship* (Sailing promotes relaxation and stress reduction like a friendship).

- **Cruise Ship** *Companionship* (Enjoying each other's company with no pressure of being in a relationship).
- **Kayak** *SoloShip* (Embracing the opportunity to be alone without feeling lonely or desiring to be in a relationship).
- **Rowing Boat:** *Partnership* (Sweep rowing requires two people both holding one oar to keep the boat balanced and moving in the same direction).

Ship Selection Worksheet

1. Which ship are you boarding?

_____

_____

_____

2. Which characteristics of that ship appeal to you?

_____

_____

_____

3. What are the limitations of the ship you've selected?

_____

_____

_____

4. How compatible is your ship with your partner's needs?

_____
_____
_____

6. What are your next steps?

_____
_____
_____

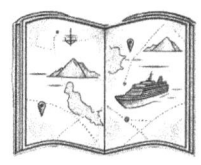 **Charter** - *Friendships, Not Clones*

Healthy relationships stem from honesty and transparency about who we really are. When we are clear about our Authentic Self and can accept all of our own assets and liabilities, we are ready to use that knowledge in relationships with others.

But the process of revealing all that we know about ourselves can feel like risky business, and rightfully so. As we experience and understand the many forms relationships can take, we must recognize that each relationship requires a different transparency formula. Our behavior with others is often situational; there is no cookie-cutter behavior that works perfectly with every person with whom we are connected. In fact, we often have unspoken rules that compel us to evaluate and define our relationships, so that we can better match our behavior with the type of relationship we are in.

For an example, here's a story about two men who have been close friends and fishing partners for several decades. When we look separately at these two, we cannot easily explain why they are even friends—but nevertheless, each feels the power and importance of the friendship.

> *Erick is an acknowledged bigot. In fact, he attests to hating virtually anyone different from himself. He doesn't focus on one race or culture or religion. They're all fair game for his negative perceptions. His language is peppered with slurs and name-calling.*

> *Steve is nearly the total opposite. He is inclusive and accepting of others, eager to learn why and how others are different. Steve works hard to exude his respect for all people, all religions, and all cultures. His dislike of others is driven by their specific behavior and not their group identity or affiliation.*

So how could these two men be friends? Let's hear what they say:

> *Steve: "It really bothers me when Erick's language is hateful and ugly. I've told him exactly how I feel when he does it. But I have never seen him hurt or wish harm on anyone. I have come to realize that his objectional behavior is purely verbal. It is just the way he talks. I have asked him not to do it when we're together and he does make an effort to do that. Whenever Erick does reject another person, it is usually due to some bad behavior he has observed that person engaging in."*

> *Erick: "Steve is OK with me, especially for a Catholic Irishman. I know he doesn't like it when I criticize other people and I guess I can see why. That's the way I talk. It's been like that all my life and gotten me in more than my share of trouble, so I have learned to scale it back a bit. But none of that has anything to do with why we are friends. We share a passionate love of the outdoors, unpopulated wilderness, clean lakes and rivers, and all of the creatures that live there. That is maybe considered our religion, but we've never said so out loud. There are very few people I am close to and Steve is near*

the top of the list. He makes me work to maintain our friendship, and nobody else in my life does that—or ever has."

So here is a friendship that is solid and lasting. It is based on one common area of interest that has managed to supersede all other differences between them. But what each has revealed to the other is carefully considered and metered out. Their love of the outdoors has served as both their safety net and their safe place where deeper communication is simply not needed. The critical point is that each person evaluates the friendship from their Authentic Self. Erick only reveals what Steve can tolerate and vice versa.

Our Authentic Self gives us the freedom and agency to choose our friends based on what works for us as individuals. As a matter of fact, once we understand ourselves, we can choose to be with others who may have a different outlook on life or an outlook that complements our own. Friendship doesn't require that everything fit perfectly: we can agree to disagree and maintain a healthy relationship because at the core of a healthy relationship is mutual respect. The fact is, we don't need to apologize for who we are; we need to understand our friendship.

Consider the groundbreaking sitcom All in the Family, in which we find bigoted husband, Archie Bunker, and his kind-hearted wife, Edith. Most would cringe at the notion of such a couple. Yet throughout the run of that sitcom, we witness the strong bond shared by the couple and that somehow their union has produced an empathetic, principled daughter, Gloria. Despite their many differences, Archie and Edith allowed one another to be authentic, and as a result, their relationship withstood the many conflicts they encountered. The moral of their story: Friendship doesn't demand assimilation but rather a respect of individuality.

The first step is the one we've already taken in this book: getting clarity on your Authentic Self. The next steps deal with what we must find in others as we develop our connection.

> **Anchors** - *Takeaways*
>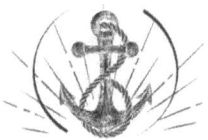
> - Whichever ship we're on, take the time to leverage what it offers.
> - Emotional safety helps to create our connection to others.
> - A healthy relationship is one in which our partner accepts us in our entirety and allows us to share our dreams and pain without fear of judgment.

Excursion 26 - Reviewing My Friendship Circle

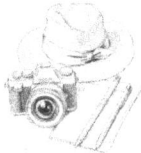

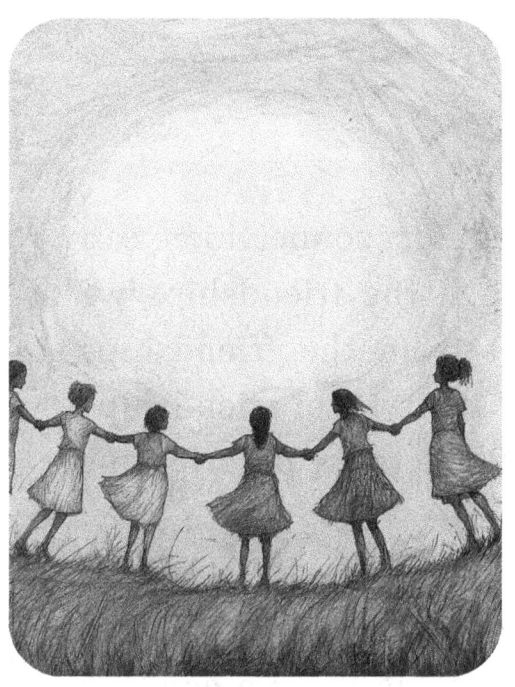

Our earlier Cruise Documents explained how mankind is born to connect with others. As we connect, we often form a friendship. Yet there are different types of friendships, which serve different purposes in our lives. For this excursion, you'll reflect on the friends in your circle, the type of friendship/purpose they represent, and any gaps that exist between the current and desired impacts of those friendships.

INSTRUCTIONS:

Step 1: Identify five to ten friends you spend the most time with or enjoy being around. Thanks to technology, these friendships may be maintained via local/in-person contact or by virtual means. Place up to five friends' initials in the box labeled CURRENT FRIENDS.

Step 2: For each of the friends you identify, categorize the type of friendship and capture that in the box labeled. If the type of friendship or person(s) cover multiple categories, select the dominant category/one that BEST characterizes the relationship. [For example, someone who is a lifelong AND convenient friend (we play cards together 2x/month) but with whom I don't share personal information, might be labeled with Activity or Lifelong in the type of friendship column, but NOT as a close Friendship].

The options are:
- Close
- Lifelong
- Activity/Convenience
- Acquaintance

Step 3: Keeping in mind that our need for connections can expand and contract over our lifespan (i.e., the friendships we established in our 20s may be different from the friendships needed in our 30s, 40s, etc.), think about the type of friendships you would like to have in your life now. Place those descriptions in the box labeled CURRENT NEEDS.

Step 4: Assess: Based on your friendship needs and the type of friendships you currently have, ask yourself, "Is there a gap?" If so, identify the friendships you want to enhance/further develop. Place that info next to the corresponding Friend it pertains to in the box labeled GAPS TO FILL.

Current Friends (up to 5)	Type of Friendship
1. Friend Initials _____	Friend #1 _____
2. Friend Initials _____	Friend #2 _____
3. Friend Initials _____	Friend #3 _____
4. Friend Initials _____	Friend #4 _____
5. Friend Initials _____	Friend #5 _____

My Current Needs (up to 5)	Gaps I Want to Fill (if any)
_____	Friend #1 _____
_____	Friend #2 _____
_____	Friend #3 _____
_____	Friend #4 _____
_____	Friend #5 _____

Step 5: Plan to address your needs. Identify ways to leverage the Healthy We portion of the model:

SHARE – How will you broach the subject with your friend? What will you say to help them understand your perspective and intentions?

ALIGN – Does your friend seem engaged/interested in the change or additional effort? If not, what is the alternative for the friendship?

PURSUE – As you move forward, how will you know your needs are getting met? What mechanisms for continuous communication will you use to ensure you and your friend(s) are moving in the same direction?

COMMIT – Does your friendship feel like it's consistently meeting your needs? Are you allowing space for yourself and your friend to remain authentic while enhancing/broadening your friendship?

FORTIFY – What ways are you keeping your friendship honest, safe, and satisfying?

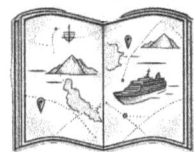 **Charter** - *Letting Your Hair Down (No hair required)*

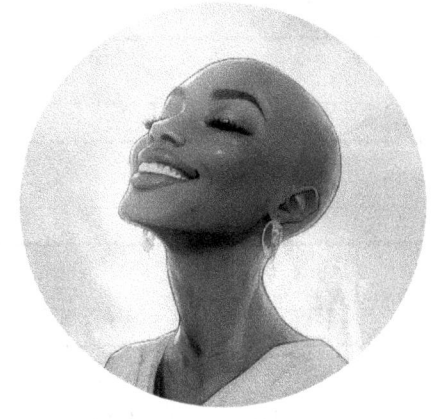

Take a moment to reflect on the craziest thing you've ever done. Who was with you at that time? Spend a few more minutes thinking about who you enjoy hanging around and why. With whom do you like spending your leisure time, and what activities do you enjoy?

> *Healthy relationships create an emotional safety that helps us to feel valued and understood.*

When we first meet a person, we typically try to be on our best behavior. Our goal (whether conscious or subconscious) is to conceal some of our deeper thoughts and beliefs that, if shared too soon, might offend them or scare them away. This is why, early in relationships, people tend to hide their idiosyncratic behaviors. For example:

> *Before they really got to know one another, she would NEVER let him see her without her makeup...and he deliberately dressed in the bathroom, afraid that his toe fungus would be a turn-off.*

In the Healthy Me portion of the workbook, we encouraged you to be REAL (Raw Expression Allows Liberation) to embrace who you are. In this Charter, we now suggest that it's time to share your realness with others—without apology. Said differently, we want you to let your hair down. While this phrase came about to represent what happens when a woman whose hair is kept tightly pinned up finally removes the pins, it has evolved to apply to anyone, whether they have hair or not. Letting our hair down means we are relaxed and authentic—no pretenses, no masks.

Healthy relationships have an abundance of trust; the individuals can remove their masks and unbind themselves.

Do you recall the first time your partner or friend saw you in a vulnerable situation? Perhaps they caught you before you were able to get your hair/nails/makeup done? Or maybe before you were able to put your partial dentures back in? Do you remember how long it took you to undress in a lighted room with your partner or to allow them to care for you while you recuperated from an illness?

Many of us feel most comfortable being ourselves with our parents and siblings because they've seen us at our worst and best, typically without judging us. Because of that familiarity we've come to trust that family will support us even when we've made poor choices or show up less than perfect.

Exposing our Authentic Self is difficult without unconditional love.

True friendship is not based on each person getting it right every time but on accepting one another with all our imperfections. When we're in a healthy SHIP, we need not question the other person's motives. There is instead an understanding that we each want the other to win and that we expect the other to bring what's good to the relationship. When such a strength-based approach exists, we're available to accept feedback from one another without being defensive. We minimize secrets so we can maintain the transparency required to build more and more trust. In essence, REALationships are emotionally safe.

10 Tips for Creating an Emotionally Safe Environment

1. **No Hidden Agendas:** Don't play mind games or be passive-aggressive with each other.
2. **For a Good Sea, See Good:** Look for the best in every situation; be slow to draw conclusions and avoid criticism.
3. **Unspoken words:** Communication can be non-verbal. Be aware of your tone and body language. Read the room, a.k.a. pay attention to how others are responding to you.
4. **Respect boundaries:** Give space as needed with no restrictions or pre-conditions.
5. **Honor priorities:** Respect what's important to others. It may mean little to you but the world to someone else.
6. **Show up:** Be consistent and do what you agreed to do; create a "no excuses" rule.
7. **Don't hit below the belt:** Expose inadequacies and/or disappointments without stockpiling them for future conflicts.
8. **Sawubona:** Help others feel seen, heard, and understood.
9. **Embrace your needs:** Confidently express what you need without conveying an apology for needing it.
10. **Grow through conflict:** Recognize that conflict provides an opportunity to learn from each other and grow our understanding of each other. Lean into conflict with a positive attitude and emerge from it with validation that your relationship is stronger than whatever the challenge encountered at that time. You have the PROOF!

Anchors - *Takeaways*

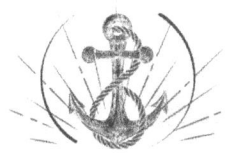

- Emotional safety encourages us to pursue individual goals without compromising our relationships.
- Trust and transparency fosters vulnerability and authenticity.
- When people genuinely like one another, they enjoy being together.

Excursion 27- Release the Bindings

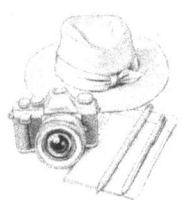

If you grew up around women who a) had long hair and b) occasionally attended formal events, you may have witnessed the arduous task of creating a bun or upsweep. These hairdos required MANY hair pins to maintain their shape throughout an event; it was common to find hair pins among the typical grooming essentials of women with long hair or hair extensions. Equally common was the complaint of women whose hair pins created discomfort due to being pinned too tightly or scratched deep into their scalps!

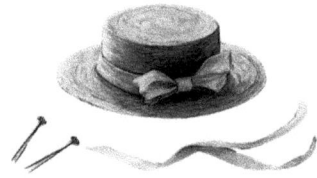

One of the most satisfying moments for a woman returning home from such an event was to remove each and every hair pin, thereby allowing their scalp to recover from the torture of being confined. While hair pinning may be a lost art, many people (this is not limited to gender nor hair length) still use imaginary pins. While they aren't literal hair pins, these habits function like pins in our daily lives. Our pins:

- Constrict our Authentic Self
- Create pinches that result in an unhealthy environment for self and others

INSTRUCTIONS: Work to identify your "hair pins". To do so, address the typical dynamics many of us use to hide our authenticity, create unnecessary conflict, and stifle sharing. If you realize there are additional pins not mentioned, simply add them to your list and consider ways to address them.

I make assumptions about others before checking-in with them.

I'll remove this PIN by:
_____

I'm only willing to see flaws in others.

I'll remove this PIN by:
_____

I use passive-aggressive cues rather than share true feelings.

I'll remove this PIN by:
_____

I overlook what others have expressed as a priority.

I'll remove this PIN by:
_____

Add your own: _____

I'll remove this PIN by:
_____

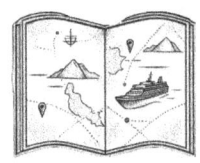 **Charter** - *Do You Know Where You're Going?*

Many people wonder if it is possible to have a healthy intimate partnership without it also being a friendship. To settle on a practical answer, let's first examine some important dynamics of friendships among lovers.

WHAT IS A FRIEND?

The following is a checklist of some key aspects of FRIENDSHIP:

- Desire to be together.
- Demonstrate love by commitment and acceptance.
- Enjoy being together.
- Together without pre-conditions.
- Feel safe with one another.
- Have fun together.
- Established over time and through experiences.
- Openly share without judgment.

At its essence, healthy friendships are based on liking and loving each other. When people genuinely like one another, they enjoy being together. When they love each other, they are together unconditionally—because of and *despite* the other's Authentic Self.

WHEN CAN'T WE BE FRIENDS?

Liking one another is NOT a key indicator to begin planning your life with some else. Despite good chemistry, there may not be enough of the key aspects cited above to move forward. Some people get excited and rush a relationship because they want physical intimacy. What they may net instead is a situationship that stunts the growth of a friendship. What's more, if not addressed honestly, such situationships can tarnish the relationship and devolve into a resentmentship!

Healthy friendships have honesty and sharing at their core, not obligation. Healthy friendships are the result of sound boundaries.

SHOULD WE BE MORE THAN FRIENDS?

So how can you tell if your friendship is ready for the next deck? Should you rely on your intuition? Do you base it on how easy it is to talk together? Going to the next level requires that we know our own destination so each of us can check our compass to determine whether we are going in the same direction. We must understand what's important to the other person and see if their priorities resonate with us.

Friendships don't require that our goals and future be in alignment, but a partnership does! We must have ties that bind us to survive the rough waters that are inevitable in life. Sharing our own direction helps the other person determine if they want to board our ship. This means we must be willing to unapologetically share our Authentic Self.

The first half of this workbook is about identifying your Authentic Self. So, the answer to "How can you tell?" is:

- Can you embrace and share who you are and where you're going?

- Is the other person clear on who they are and where they're going?
- Does your relationship reflect all those key aspects of a friendship?

If you can answer YES to everything, perhaps your friendship is ready to expand. As you answer those three bullets above, stay mindful of these typical dynamics:

- NEVER retro-fit or force-fit your desires to match someone else's path.
- Love is powerful but does NOT compensate for being on the wrong ship.
- Ensure that the other person is also clear about where they're going.
- Beware of individuals who seem invested in your plan yet have little insight about what they want. These individuals can become dependent on you without stimulating your growth.
- Some are satisfied merely watching you excel while they remain stagnant.
- There is a difference between supporting each other's goals and depending on your partner's goals!

Anchors - *Takeaways*

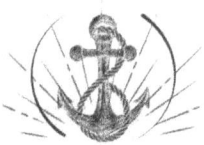

- Dishonesty can tarnish a relationship and devolve it into a resentmentship.
- Friendships don't require that our goals and future be in alignment, but a partnership does.

Excursion 28- Alignment Activity

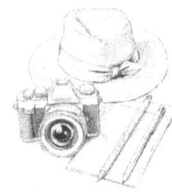

Transparency is key to individuals aligning. Without transparency, individuals may align to the wrong priorities, values, needs, goals, etc. This activity can help you clarify where you can enhance alignment to expand your relationship.

INSTRUCTIONS:

1. Write down your Authentic Self statement, which you created in Excursion 25a. Then ask the other person to share their Authentic Self statement. Take some time and discuss what's similar, what's unique, and if there are any challenges.

___

___

___

2. List your values and ask the other person to do the same. Discuss the results. Do either of you detect any red flags/potential conflicts of values?

___

___

___

3. List your priorities and ask the other person to do the same. Can you build a roadmap that will lead you to a healthy future? Often this comparison of priorities results in a common plan for the future that serves both people. For example, my priority may be to finish my college degree and by verbalizing that to my partner, we find that they had given up on a similar goal as unattainable but would love to reactivate the idea now.

_____

_____

_____

4. List your short- and long-term goals and ask the other person to do the same, even if they may not consider themselves a goal setter. Are you moving in the same direction? Identify the potential impact of the opposites on your relationship dynamics. Discuss ways to mitigate the differences and if the differences are significant enough to redefine anything about your relationship/status.

_____

_____

_____

NOTE: The process will likely reveal areas of conflict. Conflict simply means there is a gap between agreement. Such differences may require resolution. The conflict may also be an indicator of the need to RECONSIDER the healthiness of continuing to pursue the relationship. The maturity of each person will determine the health of the relationship. We must be willing to face the issues honestly.

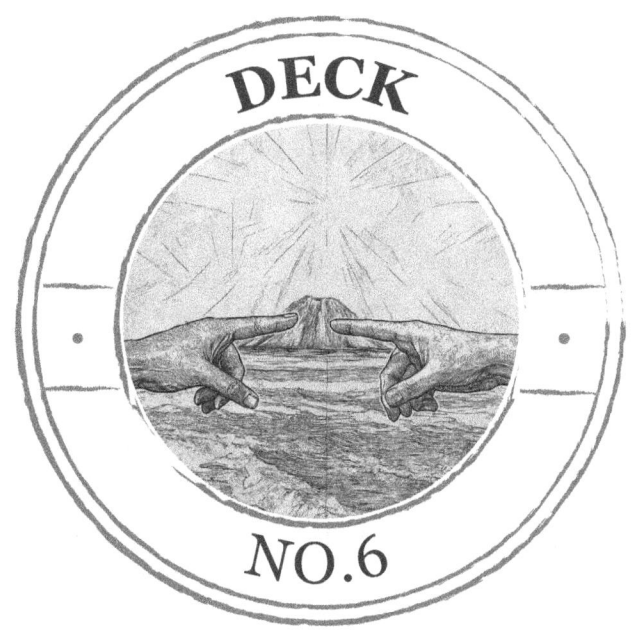

DECK 6

ALIGN DECK

If the desire to voyage together is mutual, it's critical for each of us to determine the many ways we are a good fit for one another, where there is need for enhancement, and where differences exist but don't matter enough to address. The more aligning we do, the better foundation we establish for Pursue/Commit/Fortify.

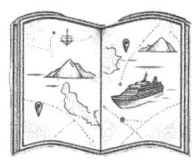 **Charter** - *So Let's Fight*

A couple that can resolve conflict in a timely and healthy way is a couple with a better chance of enjoying a healthy and fulfilling relationship. We all have experienced a honeymoon period where everything seems to be good. Many of us are not surprised by our first fight but instead we find ourselves unprepared to handle the conflict responsibly. As creatures of habit, we typically respond to conflict in a manner that we've used for past disagreements.

Since men are typically socialized to view "provide and protect" as their core relationship responsibilities, they tend toward approaching conflict from a logic/problem resolution standpoint rather than understanding how their partners are feeling. Men often, as a result, find themselves addressing the symptoms of the problem rather than the core issues/root causes. Sadly, this approach can frustrate all stakeholders, including the men, because from their perspective, the matter has been resolved. For this reason, it is quite typical for men to be heard saying, "Why does my partner keep harping on that same thing?!"

Within the general population, the answer to the above question is simple: "It's because the solution to the issue/problem was generated without you truly understanding my feelings." Women typically have a need to feel heard and validated. And they seek proof that they have, indeed, been heard and validated. Men often operate under the principle that if she is not complaining then the situation is okay until she brings it up again, hoping that the matter never resurfaces! Consequently, men can become dismissive and avoidant when dealing with conflict in their relationships. At times, the time-out solution is misused by men: they will walk away from a conflict; pretending to need time to clear their heads, but with no intentions of ever revisiting the issue. They will sometimes leave the house and return hours later hoping that their partner has magically forgotten about the conflict. Just because they're not talking about the issue doesn't mean it has been forgotten. To complicate things, men often associate make-up sex as confirmation that the matter is resolved, only to appear surprised when their partner revisits the issue during the after glow of love-making:

In the lyrics of a popular song by the Pretenders, "Thin Line Between Love and Hate," the man comes home at 5am and his partner doesn't ask him any questions while offering him warm hospitality. He misinterprets her actions, thinking that everything is okay, but in reality, it's more like: "Houston, we have a problem, and it needs to be addressed."

Men and women have been socialized to handle relationship conflicts differently. For men, the typical process is: think-resolve while skipping over "feeling". Men have been conditioned to resolve conflict without addressing emotions, having been bombarded with imagery that defines masculinity as devoid of emotions. Males, in their quest to demonstrate this masculinity, typically leave the emotional realm to females. Unfortunately, this often means that conflicts go unresolved while dysfunctional behaviors increase (e.g., infidelity, secret personal savings account, etc.), serving to mask the root causes of conflict.

Our society has conditioned men to demonstrate competitiveness and to reveal less affection. Yet intimate partnerships require them to focus on fostering a nurturing environment - one in which partners feel safe to express their feelings to resolve issues—not simply dodge problems. This means men must learn to welcome their partner's sharing their hearts, because that's when they receive the best their partner has to offer. Men must learn how to earn their partner's total transparency and to suspend their own judgment when their partner is being transparent.

In reality, most people don't want their partner walking around holding onto feelings and frustrations. In fact, if their partner can freely express their feelings, there is a better chance of resolving anything that impedes a healthy relationship. As the lyrics suggest from the indie pop song, "Say Something," when partners stop talking, they may be giving up hope that the other will do their part to help resolve the differences.

Healthy relationships are not based on winners and losers. It's possible that both people can be right in a conflict because each views things from their perspective. Unresolved conflict doesn't evaporate like morning dew. Unresolved conflict can create years of layered grievances that can be difficult to repair and endanger the future of a relationship.

Steps to resolving conflict:

1. Develop a conflict resolution plan from the beginning. The honeymoon period is the best time to establish ground rules for how conflict will be handled in the relationship. The plan should be mutual and simple to implement. Because conflict is inevitable when two or more people come together, don't wait until you have a problem to decide you need a plan. Who waits until the house is ablaze before getting insurance?!

2. Don't hide or avoid. It may be uncomfortable for you to engage in open conversation for many reasons, including past trauma and societal expectations for a person's gender role. It's critical to own your feelings. Avoiding conflict only compounds the problem while sending your partner the message that you don't care or that it's their problem, not yours.

3. Resolve quickly; don't hold on and allow things to fester or worsen.

4. Own your part of the conflict.

5. Don't try to fix your partner.

6. Don't quit until mutual resolution is declared.

7. Revisit the conversation if changes or tweaks are necessary.

8. Celebrate your success!

> **Anchors** - *Takeaways*
>
>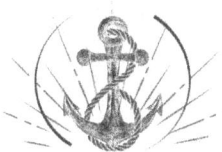
> - Conflict is inevitable.
> - Resolving conflict in a timely and healthy manner fosters a healthy and fulfilling relationship.
> - Develop a conflict resolution plan during the honeymoon period; don't wait for smoke to look for the fire extinguisher.
> - Unresolved conflict can create years of layered grievances that can be difficult to repair and which endanger the future of a relationship.

Excursion 29- Ready to Rumble...

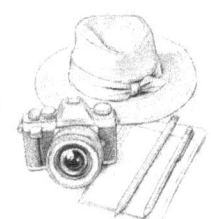

INSTRUCTIONS:

Using the eight Conflict Resolution steps in this Charter, think about the last conflict in your SHIP. Go through the steps and determine what is aligned for healthy conflict resolution as well as areas that can be improved. Identify ways to improve your response to conflict in the future.

Awareness and intentionality will help you resolve conflict more effectively.

What Works?

Which of the eight steps in the "So Let's Fight" charter are working well? Does your partner feel the same?

_____
_____
_____
_____

What Needs Work?

Which of the eight steps in the "So Let's Fight" charter do you feel would be difficult? Does your partner feel the same?

_____
_____
_____
_____

What steps can you take to strengthen your "Needs Work" items?

_____

_____

_____

_____

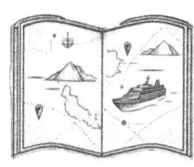 **Charter** - *Ts & Ps - Themes and Patterns*

Have you ever had a tune play on a loop in your head? What if, each time you opened the door to the refrigerator, that tune could be heard but only by you?

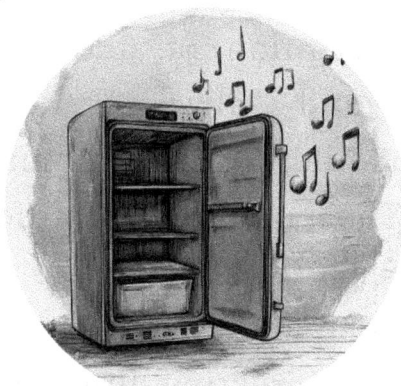

Both of those scenarios (the non-stop tune, and what happens upon opening the refrigerator) provide an analogy for the type of obstacles that keep us floundering in our relationships: themes and patterns. In our analogy, the repeating tune is the THEME, and having the tune play under predictable conditions represents PATTERNS of behavior.

If a conflict between two people goes unresolved, there is a high probability that the conflict, like a barnacle on a ship, attaches to the relationship and can be problematic. Small, seemingly unrelated actions can trigger a flare-up of such unresolved conflict caused by perceived themes & patterns (T&Ps).

Over time, partners may use T&Ps to define each other and to anticipate future actions/outcomes. Put-downs like liar, lazy, and cheater can become a staple. T&Ps become such a part of the relationship that they can be distilled down to a list of grievances that are recognizable by both parties. For example, "He always leaves the toilet seat UP!" or "She never responds to my texts when she's out with her friends." These grievances are revisited frequently to justify other behaviors or to remind our partner of their failures. If enough grievances pile up, couples can find it difficult to separate their T&Ps from the person with whom they fell in love.

This reinforcing of tainted perspectives results in discontent for both partners because they've lost sight of the "good". This occurs when we begin our description of undesirable behavior with absolutes like "never" and "always." We devolve into the complainer and the compiler, which ultimately lands us in a dynamic of avoiding. The compiler may become passive—just hoping to survive another attack—while the complainer becomes more frustrated by no perceptible change. In some cases, the compiler gives up and starts creating alternative ways to get their needs met, possibly leading to a breach in fidelity.

In other cases, the compiler starts to resist the inescapable narrative by fighting back with their own set of grievances. There is an unhealthy power component embedded in such a dynamic: The complainer takes the liberty to assess the other's motivation and (often erroneously) interprets behaviors. The outcome: the complainer seems to NOT value their partner's voice. In essence, the complainer has lost the capacity to see the "good" in their partner and has, instead, allowed the T&Ps narrative to define the relationship and imprison their partner.

So, what can be done? The answer is simple while challenging: T&Ps were created by you, so YOU have the power to change them. The Greek Pygmalion Effect provides a hint for what can be done to promote healthy outcomes:

1. Stop focusing on what's wrong and start promoting what you want. Expect good from your partner and give that person room to decide what to do.
2. Remember that the goal is not to deny or suppress our feelings and needs but to express those needs in a healthy manner and then allow your partner to decide how to respond to your needs.
3. See good, expect good, be good.
4. Use assertive communication to let your partner know what's going on with you.
5. When sharing your feelings and needs, focus on you and avoid blaming or shaming your partner. Stick to "I" statements and own you.
6. Remind yourself often of your partner's special qualities that originally caught your attention.

If you find yourself unable to move beyond the T&Ps, it's time for you to take a hard, honest look at the relationship. ASK yourself these questions: Can I see good in my partner? Is this a fulfilling relationship? Do I want to remain in this relationship?

As you formulate your answer, remember this: The goal is to be a partner in a *healthy*, fulfilling relationship.

Anchors - *Takeaways*

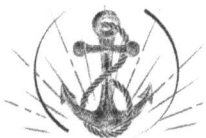

- T&Ps can be distilled down to a list of grievances that are recognizable by both parties.
- Since we create T&Ps, we have the power to change them.

Excursion 30 - Pygmalion Effect

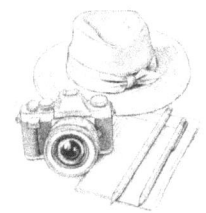

INSTRUCTIONS:

Identify grievances with your SHIP. Take note when these grievances are triggered. Find positive ways to address them. See GOOD, and look for healthy outcomes.

Grievances	Triggers	Positive Outcomes
_____	_____	_____
_____	_____	_____
_____	_____	_____
_____	_____	_____

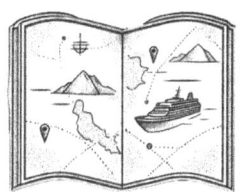 **Charter** - *Feels So Good*

Have you ever wondered why it feels so good when you first meet your partner? Everything your partner said or did seemed perfect, even if it wasn't. You were more willing to give each other the benefit of the doubt, and you viewed your relationship as a glass half-full. Do you recall all the special things you loved about your partner and what made that person so special to you? But then one day you're faced with the challenge of trying to find the good in the relationship.

Couples are able to experience this euphoric experience early in the relationship because there is not yet a counter-narrative clouding their perspective. Not until you have your first major fight do you start the process of building a conflict archive (CA) that will be used from that point to discuss problems. The CA is an archive of all the problems that weren't fully resolved and continue to crop up in future arguments.

Conflict is inevitable in a relationship. A healthy couple is not measured by whether or not they have conflict, but rather how well they navigate the *pitfalls* of conflict. Most couples never learn how to resolve conflict effectively. Unresolved conflict is like a hamster wheel that continues to turn in place, making no progress forward. Instead of feeling that warmth when we look into the eyes of our partner, we now see resentment, distrust, and confusion. Unresolved conflict serves as a barrier to happiness. These issues continue to cycle in and out of the couples' relationship, always dragging the boat to disrupt or thwart their happiness.

What can you do to hold onto that feel good experience in your relationship?

1. Destroy the CA; don't hold onto past experiences as evidence for prosecuting your case.
2. Learn how to resolve conflict quickly and effectively. Agree to have courageous conversations and remember conflict does not magically disappear just because we don't want to deal with it. Even if it goes away temporarily, that conflict will be stored in our CA, if left unresolved.
3. Reverse the conflict. Leverage the conflict as an opportunity to learn and grow; ask "What lesson did I learn from this experience?"

4. Let go and move on. It's unfair to the relationship to maintain a secret CA file cabinet; if we want to recapture the relationship, we must recreate new memories and purge the bad ones. The more we can see good in our partner, the more "good" we can feel.

Anchors - *Takeaways*

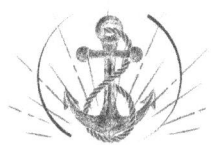

- Couples can experience euphoria early in the relationship because there is not yet a counter-narrative to cloud their perspective of each other.
- Conflict is inevitable in a relationship. A healthy couple is not measured by whether or not they have conflict, but how well the couple navigates the pitfalls of conflict.
- If a couple establishes a history of unaddressed conflict, it prevents authenticity and spontaneity, which erodes that early experience of euphoria.

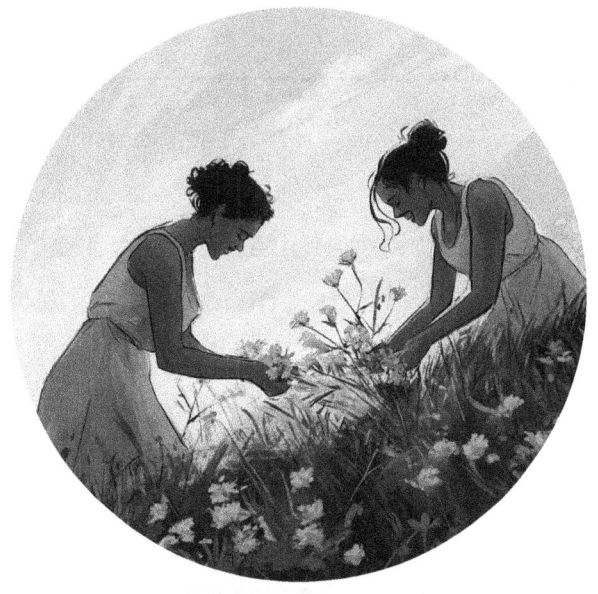

Excursion 31- Purging Your Data

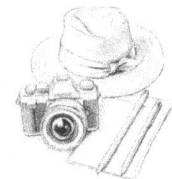

Instructions: Identify your unresolved issues and hurts. Find healthy ways to address these issues and accept the outcomes of the resolutions. Let go of any negative feelings about these experiences. If these thoughts resurface, remind yourself that these issues have been purged.

Unresolved Hurt Reminders

Review some of the items you have stored in your Conflict Archive.

These would be those arguments or disagreements that may or not be issues right now but resurface again and again in any new conflict. Select some of the "easier" items when you start.

_____

_____

_____

Resolution:

Working with your partner (or alone), determine what would be a permanent solution to the item you've stored. Understand that resolution means not revisiting the item again, so it needs to satisfy both partners.

Item 1:

_____

_____

Resolution Agreement

_____

_____

Item 2:

_____

Resolution Agreement

_____

_____

Release:

Acknowledge the removal of the resolved from your Conflict Archive. When these items resurface again (and it is likely that they will!), remind yourself and/or your partner that these have been purged and do not need to be re-negotiated.

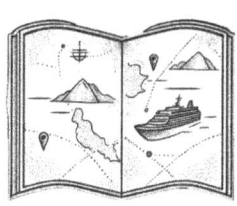 **Charter** - *Sync 2 Link*

Before we dive into the main points of this Charter, let's cover the terms "sync" and "link." If we use a dictionary definition of sync, we find that it's a shortened version of the verb SYNCHRONIZE, which means to cause two things to occur at the same time or rate.

An example of syncing occurs when a family agrees to meet up at a designated location and time before each goes off to enjoy, for instance, an amusement park. In such a situation, we might hear someone say, "Let's synchronize our watches!"

Whatever the scenario, syncing is about sameness. When we speak about syncing in a relationship, we're finding our similarities (in our values, desires, interests, needs, etc.).

Linking is simply about connecting or joining together. When we link up with others, we typically do so because there is something about the other(s) that draws us to them.

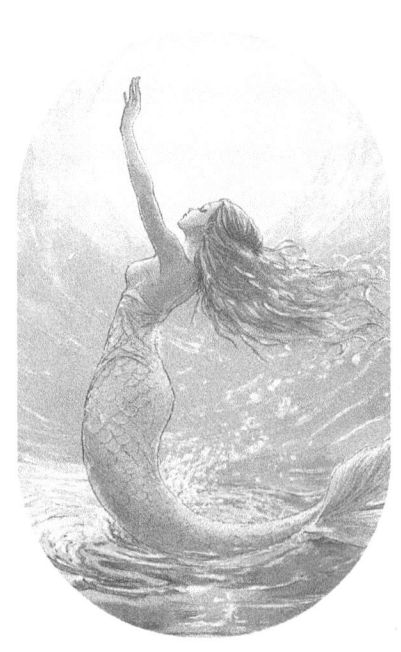

Consider Disney's 2023 live action of the The Little Mermaid. In the film, we find that despite Ariel and Eric's fundamental differences (mermaid and human, respectively), both individuals have created grottos or collections of artifacts they've gathered during their coming of age. Additionally, each has a yearning to learn more about the environments which have been rendered off limits, a situation that only serves to fuel their respective desires to break the rules and satisfy their thirst for knowledge. Their common curiosity profile activates Ariel and Eric's fate: when they meet, they have an irresistible chemistry that ultimately compels them to pursue a lifetime link to explore uncharted waters together.

Now let's think about sync and link in relation to real people and REALationships. You might have heard the phrase "opposites attract" to explain how differences can make relationships interesting. Or you may have heard that it's important for partners to have similar interests so they can stay connected. Here's the thing: both concepts can be true because there are many factors that contribute to successful, fulfilling relationships. Here are a few contributing factors to consider:

TIME: We all know of at least one couple who, after years of dating, got married; after a seemingly brief period, they then divorced. The lesson of time as a contributing factor? Time spent together does not guarantee survival of a relationship.

Time together can never be the sole indicator of the health of a relationship. Time is a QUANTIFIABLE measure that merely indicates the number of sunrises and sunsets since first linking!

CONFLICT RESOLUTION: In earlier charters, we highlighted the importance of effective conflict resolution. We emphasized the need to leverage conflicts as lessons in what's important to the other individual. Through those exchanges we get the opportunity to assess whether the other person is a good fit for who we are and what we need.

When we leverage rather than avoid conflict, we position ourselves to get clearer on our own authenticity, the authenticity of others, and the many ways we can express our needs. Conflict can actually enhance the QUALITY of our relationships if we have a healthy perspective. As a result of pursuing resolution, we can better understand one another's needs, wants, and expectations.
It's hard to explain why some relationships work while others fail. One of the most important truths to remember is to assess the ways in which your similarities and differences indicate the health of your union. Love, like the amount of time you've been together, should never be the only measure. Seek to sync in the areas that are critical for you before forging a link that may require lengthy time or enormous efforts to dismantle.

HOW SYNCHRONIZED SWIMMING MIRRORS HEALTHY RELATIONSHIPS

Synchronized swimming combines swimming, dance, and gymnastics. It requires the swimmer to have immense core strength and stamina.

Like us, each individual in the relationship should understand their Authentic Self and show resilience while aligning for a Healthy We . Many SHIPS fail because inadequate time is spent on alignment and too much value is placed on initial feelings and desired destinations/outcomes.

Most synchronized swimmers can hold their breath for about three minutes since the swimmers are underwater for most of the performance.

To really understand another person, we must go beneath the surface. The more time we spend under the surface, the better we will be able to be in sync in the future. Some folks treat relationships like buying a used car; they only want to focus on the exterior while spending very little time under the hood.

Special technology is used in competition to allow the swimmers to hear the music underwater without damaging their hearing.

When we get under the surface, we must avoid getting lost in our partner's past while also understanding it as we decide how best to proceed.

Synchronized swimming teams practice more than any other sport. They average 8-10 hours per day for six days of the week.

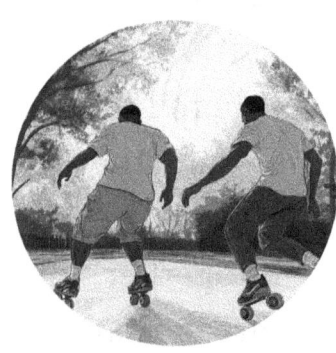

There is no fast track for aligning with one another, so take care to not link prematurely. That's why dating is so important. The more time spent together and sharing experiences with one another, the more opportunities to get below the surface and evaluate what we're getting. The goal is NOT perfection but instead healthy. There may be scar tissue from old wounds but what's important is that the individual has gone through the healing process. We are not afraid of past mistakes; but rather, we are concerned about mistakes that are unaddressed.

Anchors - *Takeaways*

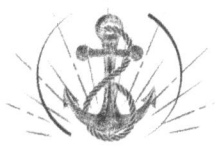

- Syncing is about sameness, and linking is about connecting or joining together.
- Time together can never be the sole indicator of the health of a relationship.
- Sync in critical areas before forging a link that could require enormous efforts to dismantle.
- The more time we spend under the surface, the better we're capable of future syncing.

Excursion 32 - Sync 2 Link Activity

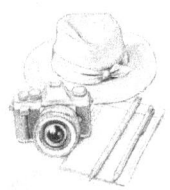

Listed below are topics that you may want to explore as you decide how to proceed on the commitment deck. Determine if you and your partner are aligned on each topic by indicating a + for similar and − for different. If you're different, that's okay! This opens a conversation. In discussing it, were you able to come to an understanding? Mark Yes/No in the outcome column. A "NO" indicates an area that needs more attention.

Topics	Similar/Different	Outcome
Finances		
Extended Family		
Children		
Culture/Faith		
Intimacy		
Resolving Conflict		
Friends		
Geographical Location		
Goals		
Other		

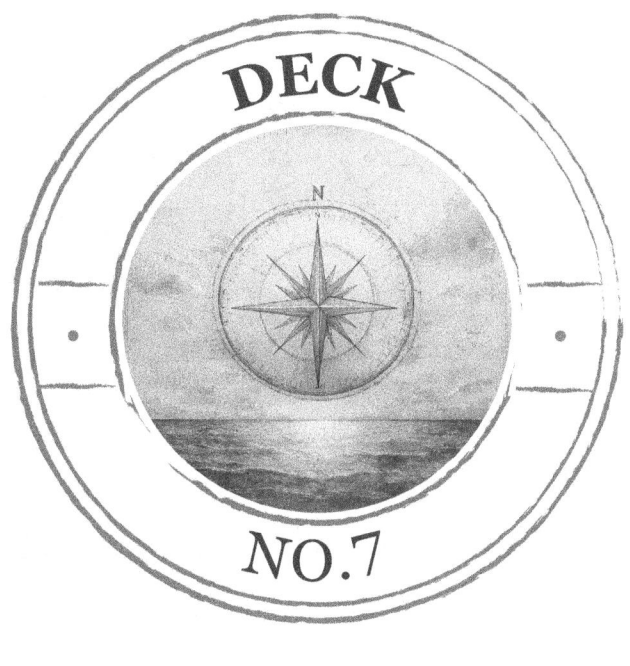

DECK 7

PURSUE DECK

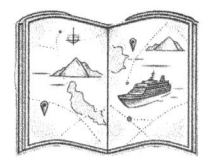 **Charter** - *The Great Pursuit: Not an Eclipse*

In the 1997 hit movie Soul Food, Teri and Miles are a power couple—they're both attorneys. As Teri advances her career at the firm, Miles is much more interested in pursuing his passion for music. This different pursuit frustrates Teri, who feels that Miles is squandering both money and his law degree by pursuing this hobby. Miles wanted Teri to embrace his love for music, and the fact that they aren't on the same page creates tension in their marriage and ultimately causes the demise of their relationship.

How does the movie Soul Food compare to real life? Simply put: It's important that a couple agrees on their priorities. As you prepare to commit to another person, understand that the commitment is about coming together to form a healthy partnership. Such a process requires collaboration and compromise—without them, you'll likely have a shipwreck.

Where do two well-meaning people begin?

First, let's think about each person as a whole—one is a Sun, and the other is a Moon. Each has their own purpose and goals. In relationships, each party has their own purpose and goals, too. When two people decide to create a Healthy We , it's critical that they share values and interests to determine where there is commonality.

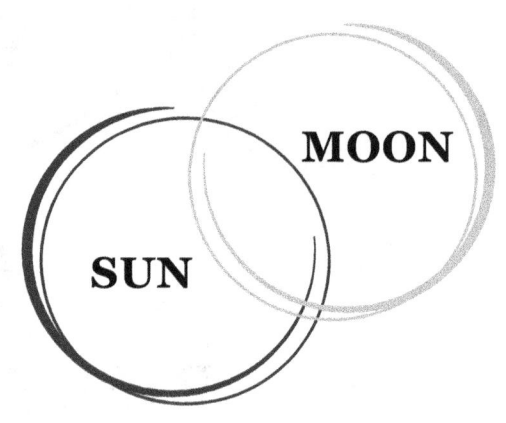

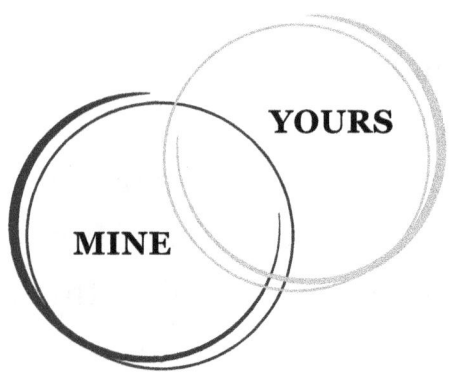

Each party brings their Authentic Self to the experience; it's important that neither is made to sacrifice nor subordinate their Authentic Self/Healthy Me. Instead, they should identify where there is overlap so the Healthy We /partnership can build from there. Consider the diagram to the left, which represents two people who have found the common areas where their values/interests overlap. This shared space is a good place to establish priorities for the relationship.

Remember: Pursuing priorities is a partial eclipse like the diagram and NOT like a total eclipse! Healthy We signifies that one partner does not overshadow or block the other partner but rather that partners work together toward mutual goals and to address differences in their priorities/goals. Healthy We means neither dominates the other nor treats their partner's purpose/goals as inferior. When Healthy We exists, we find ways to discuss and find agreements about how we'll handle what lies beyond the overlap.

Challenging...But Well Worth It!

Healthy We is not an easy achievement. Because it is an ongoing pursuit, there will likely be times that you question why you ever embarked on this journey! Here are a few key insights to revisit whenever you doubt your efforts' worthiness compared to the prize:

- Revisit your priorities frequently and make changes as needed.
- Recall how hard you pursued each other when you first met. Bring that same energy to sustain your Healthy We !
- Healthy relationships have a direction. The partners adjust and move as if dancers. Remember Fred Astaire and Ginger Rogers? Their renowned partnership as dancers was the result of demonstrating grace and agility as they moved as one. Each had their own part, sometimes at opposite sides of the dance floor, but they always had the same outcome in mind.
- Avoid a shutdown which can impair established connection. Instead pursue Healthy We to gain clarity and proceed with confidence.

As we explore and identify the priorities that we each bring to the REALationship, keep in mind that each partner will have different priorities. For example, let's say one partner has a passion for wardrobe design and has a part time job in a dress shop, while the other has a passion for writing. Both are important passions, but only to the partner who has that passion. When they explain their priority to each other, they realize that each one ultimately brings them satisfying opportunities to help others. It doesn't matter if the writer cares, individually, about wardrobe design; the writer needs to care about it because their partner cares. In that discussion they find that the overlap of helping others makes their REALationship stronger.

Anchors - *Takeaways*

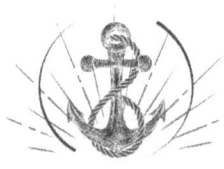

- Healthy We signifies that one partner does not overshadow or block the other partner but rather that partners work together toward mutual goals and to address differences in their priorities/goals.
- Healthy relationships have a direction. The partners adjust and move as dancers.
- Remember how hard you pursued each other when you first met. Bring that same energy to sustain Healthy We !

Excursion 33 - Commonalities: Dance of the Sun & Moon

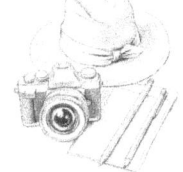

Isn't it heartwarming to see a couple take to the dance floor and appear so connected and fluid? There are even fun events which pair complete strangers to swing dance together, as if they've been choreographed partners for years! The secret to a winning combination is trust in self and a willingness to communicate with your partner. Think about it: in dance, the only language is non-verbal; watching your partner and responding to the requests that are expressed by how the partner holds your hand(s).

Seeing such coordination and competence is inspiring because the couple achieves excellence together without losing their individuality. It's very much how the sun and moon share the sky as they continuously achieve their purpose yet maintain their uniqueness. They just seem to dance!

For this excursion, you'll work with your partner to identify areas where you can prioritize aspects of your shared life that overlap yet could benefit from you and your partner being intentional to achieve a fluid dance.

STEP 1: Each partner creates their own list of values and interests (e.g., a value might be creating a shared savings account for vacations; an interest might be learning to play golf).

STEP 2: Partners compare their personal lists of values and interests to identify where there may be COMMON items (e.g., in making a comparison, Joe & Joan realize that they are both interested in learning to play a sport).

STEP 3: Partners discuss how to handle that which is important to each BUT is not on the other partner's list (e.g., DIFFERENCES between Joan & Joe are that Joe would like to get a graduate degree. Joan has no interest in an advanced degree. They discuss ways Joan can be supportive of Joe's interest, which include picking kids up from afterschool programs on days Joe has class).

REPEAT: Invite one another to "dance" periodically to ensure no external influences have altered earlier priorities/approaches. If such has occurred, let the dance begin again!

Partner 1

1.
2.
3.
4.

Partner 2

1.
2.
3.
4.

Partnership Priorities

1.
2.
3.
4.

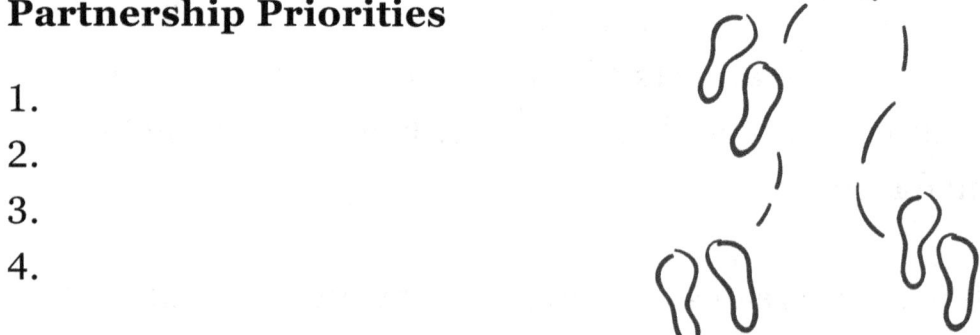

PURSUE There will always be differences in outlooks, skills, priorities, backgrounds, and countless other facets—none of us are clones, nor must we be. What's most important is for us to maintain our Authentic Selves as we make the journey together.

For ours to be a successful, happy, healthy voyage, we must have common pursuits in addition to our individual pursuits. It's not enough to be aware of the ways we align—we must ensure that we're both chasing what we determine to be important. If aligning only nets lip service from one member of the crew while the other member does all the work of PURSUE, the likelihood for a shipwreck is high.

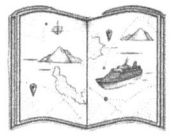 **Charter** -*Needs, Wants, and Expectations— What's The Difference and Why Does It Matter?*

Let's first explore the terms to better understand how to apply the knowledge relating to Healthier ME and WE.

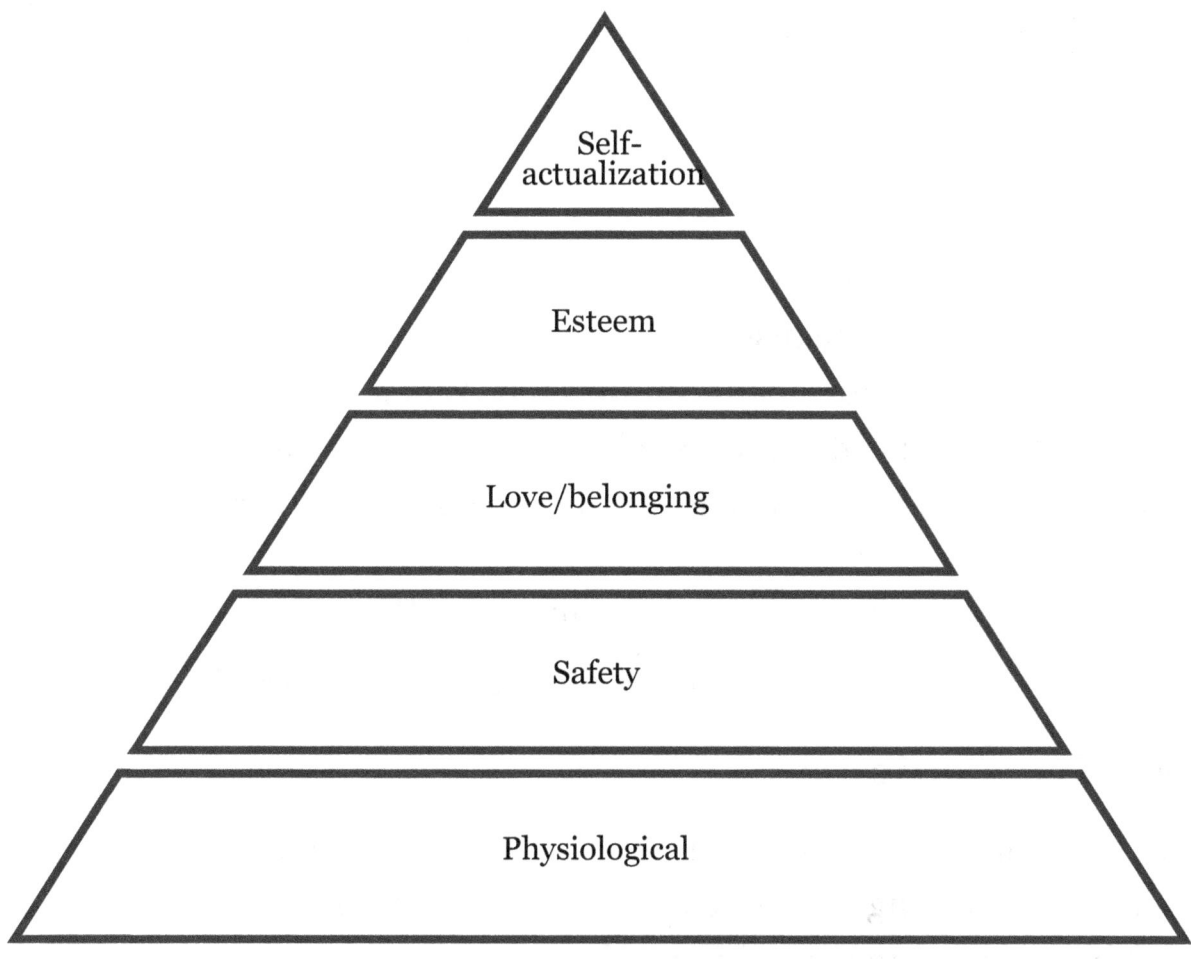

About Needs:

In 1943, Abraham Maslow created a motivational theory pyramid to help people better understand human motivation. The pyramid illustrates that our base (or basic) needs are related to survival—or said slightly differently—we need that which contributes to our physical and mental health. Without food, shelter, clothing, etc., we would perish.

As you move up the pyramid, our needs get more complex, but the essence of Maslow's theory is that we are motivated to satisfy our most basic needs FIRST before we worry about or pursue higher-level needs. So, the next time you think about your needs, ask yourself, "Is this something that contributes to my overall HEALTH and ability to survive?

About Wants:

A "want" is a desire or a yearning. No matter how deeply we may yearn for a 12-room house, yearning doesn't transform our want to a "need" because a 1-room shack can also provide the shelter necessary for health or survival. When you compare the attainment of needs and wants, however, the feelings they produce within us helps us to distinguish between them:

- Fulfilling needs results in better HEALTH
- Fulfilling wants allows us to experience HAPPY

About Expectations:

As implied in the root of the word, to EXPECT means that we believe something is due, coming, going to occur, or imminent (often referring to something welcome or pleasant). Because we are usually eagerly anticipating whatever it is when we have expectations, the greater the joy we attach to our expectation being met, the deeper the disappointment can be when the expectation is not met. For example, a youth approaching a milestone birthday for which the parents have hinted that they're planning a HUGE gift. If the youth eagerly anticipates that gift to be a car and, instead, receives tickets to the local movies, the disappointment would (understandably) be tremendous. How tremendous? As tremendous as the elation would have been to receive the car!

The irony of expectations is that many of us expect others to know what we expect! That's asking others to be clairvoyant or "mind-readers" of our beliefs. Simply put, it's grossly UNFAIR.

What do needs, wants, and expectations (NWE) have to do with Healthy Me and Healthy We?

Recall that Healthy Me is a lifetime pursuit to understand and bring your Authentic Self to all relationships. Your NWE are components of your Authentic Self and as such are included with what is to be known, owned, and (appropriately) shared by you with others. Yet if you aren't clear about what is vital to your health, happiness, and harmony among others, you're set up for ongoing stress and strife. The stress: from the dissatisfaction of fulfilling needs and wants that are not authentically yours. The strife: from the constant conflict that lurks like an undercurrent, ready to swell and capsize the vessel, when unvoiced expectations are not met.

What can I do about it? —HINT: There are NO Quick Fixes!

Most people know what they want but don't take the time to share their NWE with others. Remember: people are not mind-readers and may not fully understand your NWE unless you share it with them. It's also important to keep in mind that our

NWE can change as we go through the life cycle. It's therefore even more important to maintain open communications with those you deem significant in your life—open communications regarding your NWE, as they evolve. A Healthy Me develops the capacity to adjust and accommodate others as personal clarity about self and others occurs.

Excursion 33 - Healthy, Happy, and Harmony

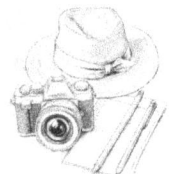

In his Hierarchy of Needs, Maslow suggests that if our basic needs are not met, it's difficult for us to pursue higher-level needs like the need to be happy. For this activity, let's think about NEEDS, but reframe needs with a bit more precision: Needs are what is required for you to be HEALTHY. Remember, healthy doesn't mean "perfect and flawless," but rather what's necessary for there to be balance, stability, and/or a sense of equilibrium.

Instructions

Part 1: Read each question and give it your honest response

A. What do I need to be healthy?

_____

_____

_____

_____

B. Am I taking responsibility for tending to my needs?

_____

_____

_____

_____

C. Am I relying on others to tend to my needs?

_____

_____

_____

_____

D. In past friendships or relationships, did I compromise my needs to accommodate someone else? Did that choice produce good results for me?

_____

_____

_____

_____

PART II. Use the list of CONSIDERATIONS on the next page to remind yourself about the importance of NWE to your personal Health and the health of your REALationships. You may choose to create memes or prompts for yourself by putting each on a Post-It or other format that can be placed on a mirror, in your handbag, or a daily pop-up message within your mobile device. Whatever it takes to sustain the use of as many of the considerations as possible.

Considerations

- The difference between a need and want is that needs met result in HEALTHY while wants achieved allow us to experience HAPPY.

- We may not get everything we want but it's important to share our wants with those around us.

- Wants can change more frequently than needs but they are important to sustain the joy in relationships.

- Needs foster security while wants facilitate happiness.

- Happiness reinforces pursuit of our passions and interests. The "pursuit of happiness" is a cornerstone phrase of the U.S. Constitution to which we all have a right.

- Wants highlight our uniqueness and represent the key features of our "special sauce."

- Expectations expressed bring clarity to relationships and serve to minimize conflict.

- Clear expectations facilitate harmony in relationships because each knows what the other may eagerly desire while also reducing opportunity for misunderstandings. Many fail to invest the time to express their expectations and default to build their relationships on assumptions.

- Relationship history has proven that much intimate conflict stems from the failure to spell out what partners expect from one another. For example, while dating a couple did not talk about the distribution of household chores. However, once they moved in together, one partner assumed that the chores would be equally shared while the other partner thought taking out the trash each week was adequate. Over time, the couple was struggling, and communication broke down--creating resentment. All of this due to expectations which were not discussed before moving forward in the relationship.

- Discomfort in discussing your expectations is an indication that you may require more work on Healthy ME and Healthy We (the REALationship). Expectations are a component of what gets shared by Healthy.

- NWE is a powerful tool/approach to help create health, happiness, and harmony in your relationships. Invest time to evaluate if something is missing in your NWE.

- Are you pursuing Healthy and Happy now? If not, START TODAY!

Anchors - *Takeaways*

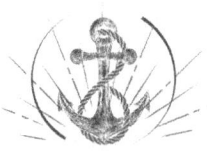

- Fulfilling NEEDS helps us achieve health while fulfilling WANTS allows us to experience happiness.
- Knowing the difference between our needs and wants positions us for better understanding of ourselves AND for better communication of them to others
- Don't expect others to understand you/your needs if you don't. Your work is to understand your own needs; and your responsibility is to help others to understand your needs by expressing them.

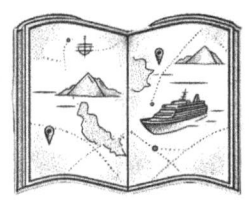

Charter - *The Shutdown*

The shutdown is an unhealthy tactic couples use when they are unhappy with each other. It occurs when one partner chooses not to engage with the other. The shutdown is a learned behavior that is deployed when one feels angry or hurt. One or both partners decide to stop communicating, thereby interrupting the FLOW of the relationship. Most shutdowns are accompanied by a guessing game that requires the other partner to figure out what disrupted the FLOW.

IMPACT – The shutdown can be a frustrating process because it forces one partner to mind-read in order to resolve the conflict. If the shutdown is not addressed swiftly, it can linger for days—sometimes weeks—while each partner sits waiting for the other to blink. The shutdown can be triggered anytime; it brings to the surface old wounds and unresolved issues. The person who initiates the shutdown—the shut-downer—typically feels justified for pulling the rug out from under the relationship. Yet it's difficult to conduct a rational conversation with the shut-downer because their emotions are driving their decision-making process. What's more, the shutdown does not resolve the issue, but instead exacerbates the problem and leaves both parties even more resentful and injured. During the shutdown, the shut-downer often renders themselves unavailable to process their feelings, ultimately holding out for the other person to learn the lesson of "Don't mess with me." Shutdowns are destructive and erode the feel-good aspect of relationships. If they regularly occur, the couple gets used to the tactic and they grow further and further away from each other.

REMEDY - What can you do to avoid using, or being victimized by, a shutdown? Here are a few approaches:

1) Own your feelings. Avoid turning inward when you are hurt. Speak out and help your partner understand your feelings. Use an assertive voice and share your truth.

2) Be realistic and try to remember that you may not be able to resolve all issues right away. The mere sharing of your thoughts with your partner initiates the healing process. It may take time to work through the complexities of the conflict.

3) Take care to avoid exaggeration. Express what is necessary, then let go and move on.

4) Push yourself to bring whatever you are harboring out into the open—don't let it fester inside. Problems are difficult to resolve if they stay hidden or buried.

5) Ask yourself the question: Is this an issue I can resolve on my own, or do I need my partner's involvement? If so, I can express my feelings such that I am heard/understood, and afterwards I move on. Doing this keeps you from shutting down and zapping the positive energy out of the relationship.

6) The next time you are inclined to shut down, remind yourself that on the other side of that negative behavior is someone you love.

7) Never allow the day to end with a shutdown—it makes for mutually uncomfortable bedfellows!

Anchors - *Takeaways*

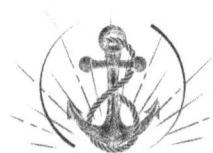

- Shutting down is a learned behavior when one feels angry or hurt.
- Don't let feelings fester.
- Never let the day end with a shutdown.

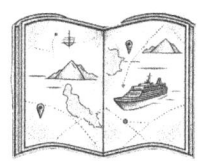 # Charter - *F.L.O.W.*

"Happiness is when what you think, what you say, and what you do are in harmony."
~ Mahatma Gandhi

There is a traditional and time-honored practice from ancient China called Feng Shui (pronounced fung shway) whose purpose is to create harmony between individuals and their surrounding environment. The literal translation of Feng Shui is "wind-water;" it is practiced by ensuring that one's surroundings are designed, furnished, and decorated in a manner that allows energy to flow freely.

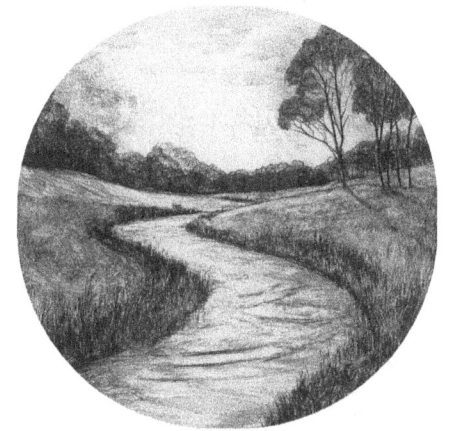

Simply put: to flow, energy cannot be blocked. For example, for sunlight to flow freely through a window, the window must be clean; for air to flow freely through a room, the vents cannot be blocked. Think of Feng Shui/wind-water as shorthand for "able to flow."

Feng Shui is also important in relationships. For relationships to be healthy, each person's authentic energy must be allowed to flow. When a person's energy is flowing freely, they spend less time wearing a mask that blocks their true self. Additionally, partners acknowledge and accept one another. This means no lies and no deception but instead truth and transparency, like sunshine through a window or air circulating through a room.

So how can a couple work to achieve that flow in their

relationship? First let's identify the typical dynamics that exist when a relationship lacks flow. In these relationships, challenges and conflicts are typically handled in a dysfunctional manner, resulting in few displays of compassion, empathy, or the proverbial benefit of the doubt as problems arise.

Since relationships only thrive when both parties want it to work, the most important preliminary action is to ensure that the relationship is not one-sided. When one of you is not committed to the work, the relationship can't flow.

With commitment, the real work of creating truth and transparency begins. An easy way to understand and remember the effort for FLOW is:

First Listen, then Own your Work

FLOW is a choice to work through challenges without blaming or demonizing your partner. Unfortunately, couples often build their relationship on a weak foundation; each brings into their new relationship their past negative experiences, which form a wall that blocks FLOW.

The nature of FLOW acknowledges that all relationships have challenges, but healthy relationships are composed of partners who choose to perceive challenges as opportunities to enhance the relationship. Applying FLOW allows partners to navigate the small issues so they don't snowball into larger issues. Instead, they are able to put life's events into perspective and respond to situations based on what's most important. Applying FLOW allows partners to address those important issues while being reminded of their partners' beauty—all the reasons they were originally smitten!

How to increase the FLOW in your relationship:

1. **Validate your choice:** FLOW can only happen when you are committed to your partner. If you find yourself wondering if this is the right person, you owe it to yourself and your partner to determine what you want before you move forward.
2. **Prioritize:** Avoid fussing over the little stuff. When asked, many couples can't even remember the initial trigger of an argument. What's more, they are typically embarrassed to acknowledge the silly/petty issue that began a conflict.
3. **Extinguish the Small Fires:** Most raging infernos begin as tiny sparks. FLOW means that neither partner is playing mind games or holding grudges. Remember: Wind and water make contact but keep moving—and so should you. Address the issue head-on, then move on.
4. **Seek the Message:** Every situation provides an opportunity to learn and grow. Stop fighting long enough to LISTEN and sift through what you hear to learn, work, and grow.
5. **Carpe Diem:** Seize the opportunity to increase FLOW! Each of us only gets one life; any day you live without FLOW is a day you've lost a chance to contribute to your peace and happiness.

Anchors - *Takeaways*

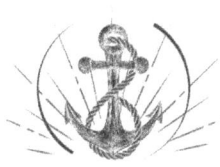

- FLOW is a choice to work through challenges without blaming or demonizing your partner.
- Relationships can only thrive when both parties want it to work.
- Every situation provides an opportunity to learn, work, and grow.

Excursion 34 - My FLOW

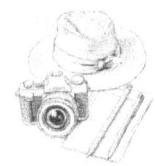

Get started by asking yourself--

- Am I flowing with my partner right now?
- When was the last time I experienced FLOW in a relationship?
- What's blocking my FLOW?

Flow Worksheet

1. How will you know when you have achieved flow with a partner, or within a group? What do you need to have flow?

_____

_____

_____

2. Can you experience flow if your partner does not? How, why, when?

_____

_____

_____

3. What can you do within a relationship to make flow more available to you or to others? What steps can you take to maintain the flow you have already experienced?

_____

_____

_____

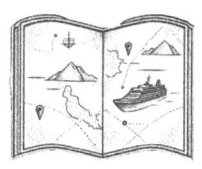 **Charter** - *Shipwreck*

What is an intimate partnership "shipwreck? If it happens, can it be repaired? As the term suggests, a shipwrecked intimate partnership is one that has suffered damage. For our purposes, we'll use the nickname relationshipwreck.

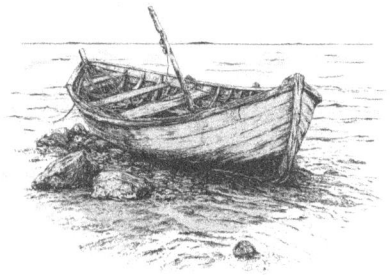

There are many causes for damage which include, but aren't limited to, infidelity, an inability to manage blended family challenges, or addiction. Staying with this analogy, in a relationshipwreck, the captain bears the burden of restoring the ship's C-Worthiness. By C-Worthy, we mean that the relationship is worthy of commitment.

Once damage has occurred, deciding how to address it becomes the central challenge. Is it more cost effective to take the loss and file a claim (divorce or separation)? If so, should you look for a new vessel or just retire from the sea for good? Do you make critical repairs because of the sentimental value of the vessel and your unwillingness to let it go?

A relationshipwreck isn't necessarily the end. It could, in fact, mark a new beginning with parts that are both new and improved. Before either repairing or abandoning a relationshipwreck, ask yourself these questions:

Do I see good in my partner? In intimate partnerships, the inability to see and acknowledge the other person's goodness has been labeled contempt by psych experts. In this piece, we'll refer to such relationshipwreck dynamics as hostility characterized by one or both partners' inability to see any positive in the other. These relationshipwreck interactions are fueled by mutual disdain where the glass is always half empty. To declare the vessel a C-Worthy REALationship, there must be MORE desire to see the other partner win than a personal desire to be right.

Do I enjoy being around this person? Fun is an important ingredient to any healthy relationship. Couples tend to experience fun during the friendship phase of relationships but fail to nurture levity and kindness once they transition to a companionship or intimate partnership.

How bad is the damage? In an actual shipwreck, the damage is usually below the surface. It cannot be repaired while the ship is still in the water. Is this the way your relationship is going? Are you hanging on because you love how it felt before? Can you actually fix the damage and remain afloat? Is your partner willing to do that work?

Do I feel safe and secure around my partner? Safety and security are the two pillars of a healthy REALationship. Safety means being both vulnerable and authentic around the other person without them judging or ridiculing you. Being accepted allows partners to remove anything that masks their authenticity. Security is assurance that despite adversity, the other person will always throw a life line. Safety and security engender the confidence each has in the other while both work to maintain the C-Worthiness of the REALationship.

Anchors - Takeaways

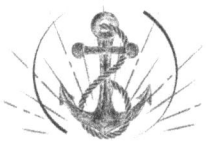

- A relationshipwreck could mark a new beginning with new and/or improved aspects.
- Declaring your ship C-Worthy (commitment worthy) means there's MORE desire to see the other partner win than a personal desire to be right.
- Requirements to avoid relationshipwreck: we can both see good in the other, we enjoy being around each other, and we feel safe and secure with one another.

Excursion 35 - Relationshipwreck

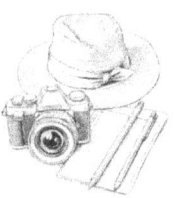

At some point during its journey, every SHIP will face adversity. This is especially true when priorities are being established during Pursue. During this portion of the journey, it's important to address challenges and choices. If they're handled well, we're able to strengthen our SHIP; if mishandled, we can cause a relationshipwreck.

Some incidents are repairable in the water, while other situations require dry docking. In the upcoming fortify deck, you will be working with the INWI excursion, which reminds us that not every relationshipwreck requires the same response. In that excursion, we identify four distinct responses to relationshipwrecks:

- **It's Not Worth It (INWI)** - Things that can be resolved with minimal intervention.
- **Game Changer** - Incidents that must change over time (non-emergencies that are serious enough to warrant some changes).
- **Game Over** - Situations where there is zero tolerance for that behavior.
- **Must Haves** - What each partner requires to maintain a healthy relationship.

This excursion will provide information you can reference when you get to the fortify deck

INSTRUCTIONS:

I. Complete the activity below using the outline identifying your most recent relationshipwrecks. Identify its impact on you and others and the lessons you learned from those experiences.

II. Once you've captured the type of relationshipwrecks, their impacts, and lessons learned, take a step back to determine if there are patterns within these incidents. (e.g., lack of communication, no follow-through on commitments, blaming partner when things go poorly, etc.)

III. As a final step, try to identify ways you might be able to resolve these issues.

Capture your info in the table below.

Type of Relationshipwreck	Impact of Relationshipwreck	Lessons Learned

Complete this sentence after reviewing the relationshipwrecks captured in the table above:

"Upon reflection, I notice there is a pattern. The pattern seems to be _____

_____

_____

Capture your info in the table below.

Ideas for Resolving Negative Impact	Ideas for Applying Lessons I Learned

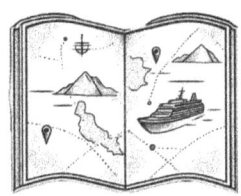

Charter -*Buyer's Remorse*

Have you ever made a large purchase and later questioned it? Unlike retailers who give buyers time to return a purchase without penalty, relationship decisions can have lifelong consequences. It is therefore important to count the cost before we make the commitment to move forward with a relationship.

Because it's difficult to fully know that a person will be a good partner unless we invest the time to understand what we want or who we are, this workbook started with Healthy Me —empowering you to make decisions that fit your life purpose. How many friends and/or family members have you heard exclaim "I knew I shouldn't have married this person; all the signs were right in front of me?"

As you complete the Pursue Deck, you have an opportunity to identify your priorities and discuss them with your fellow shipmate. Take care to not force the relationship when there are signs suggesting you should abort the mission. It's like trying to fit a square peg into a round hole: With enough force, the square peg will fit, but there will be no room for growth and adjustment. What results is one partner feeling stuck. There are no guarantees that a relationship will work even after we have done a thorough inspection of the SHIP. However, if we make careful decisions by considering each person's priorities, we may reduce relationship hardships.

At this stage of the voyage, you may find yourself in between a status, with not enough momentum to move forward as an intimate partnership, but "in" too much to let go. Here's a typical dynamic of the in-between status:

> *We have invested time and resources in the relationship and may be sensitive to public opinion. We might have met our shipmate's family and friends; many are expecting that we're moving to the Commit Deck. Despite expectations, however, we may know that there is something missing or troubling us, but that missing something may be offset by some qualities on our wish list. We may conclude that the shipmate is not too bad.*

Some advice for those who feel in-between: Before you go to the next deck, ask yourself, "Can I live with what's missing, assuming that my partner will not change?"

In 1991, the British band Clash reached the top of the UK charts with the hit, "Should I Stay or Should I Go?" This rock song wrestles with relationship indecision. The lyrics suggest that either decision will be difficult to make, which is why it's important to be clear with your shipmate your intentions.

Being in-between can skew our ability to make sound decisions. Just remember: Accepting some pain today can avoid catastrophic pain in the future.

Anchors - *Takeaways*

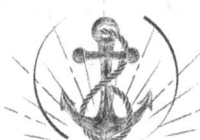

- Relationship decisions have long-term consequences.
- Make decisions that fit your life purpose.
- Board the right SHIP with the right shipmate.
- Determine if you are in-between or merely settling to avoid a painful future.

Excursion 36 - In-between Assessment

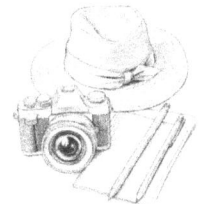

Before you venture to the Commit Deck, you should decide whether this is the right time and person. There can be multiple factors involved in this decision, such as age, career, cultural expectations, and unresolved trauma. Remember: We are striving for healthy, not perfect. You may not get everything you want, but you must be confident that you are connecting with someone who is committed to Healthy Me. With that in mind, listed below are important factors to consider in moving forward.

INSTRUCTIONS: There are two columns, Commit and Let Go. If you feel that the factor along the left has been addressed (and you feel good about it), place it in the Commit column. If not, place it in the Let Go column. After you have considered all the factors, write a statement about why you should stay or go.

Factors:	**Commit**	**Let Go**
Values		
Priorities		
Goals		
Family		
Fun		
Conflict Resolution		
Money		
Interpersonal Skills		
Connection		
Attraction		
Should I Stay or Should I Go?		

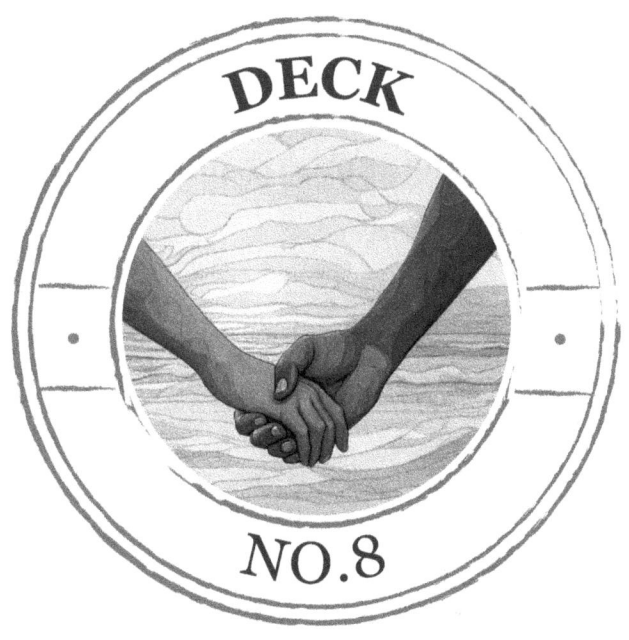

DECK 8

COMMIT DECK

COMMIT may sound simple and straightforward, but it's often difficult. Why? Could it be faulty memories on both individuals' parts, each remembering different priorities? Or maybe competing priorities allow one or both partners to lose sight of their original plans? Whatever the reason, none of us is the exact same person we were just yesterday, and slight changes over time can veer us off our original course. Think about how easily gaining or losing just one or two pounds per month can impact your wardrobe!

The key of Commit is to stay focused on what was mutually determined to be important. Revisit those priorities and original mindsets to ensure engagement levels are still mutually high. Apply the adage: "We can never step into the same river twice" as a reminder that everything changes, even the priorities we established when we first embarked. Commit means being intentional about revisiting and, if necessary, reestablishing priorities throughout the voyage.

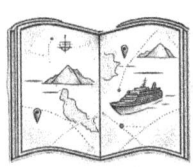 **Charter** - *Why We Stay*

Why we stay in our relationships can be a complex and personal decision. We have probably all heard the many reasons why people remain in unhealthy relationships:

- It's cheaper to keep her.
- I see potential.
- I know my partner will change once we have the baby.
- I am afraid to be alone.
- I'm damaged goods. Who'll want me now?
- I'm over the hill.
- I made my bed so I have to lay in it.
- My faith dictates that I hang in there.
- I'm doing it for the children.
- I don't want to give up my lifestyle.

This charter is written without judgment of others. We are the ultimate decider of what is best for us. That said, NO ONE should remain in an abusive relationship. Intimate partner violence is serious, illegal, and should be handled carefully and with a trained professional. It may seem obvious to advise a victim to leave an abusive relationship, but leaving is the riskiest time for survivors who might be hurt—or, even worse, killed. If you are living in fear or have been abused, seek support from local domestic violence resources. Remember, you are not alone, and you deserve to be in a healthy and safe relationship.

As you seek to establish healthy relationships, keep in mind that you are not looking for Mr. or Ms. Perfect. The goal is to have a strong emotional connection with your partner where you work toward mutual goals, have fun being together, and learn from each other. Each relationship has seasons; there will be times of great accomplishments and memory-making, while other times you may feel exhaustion and defeat.

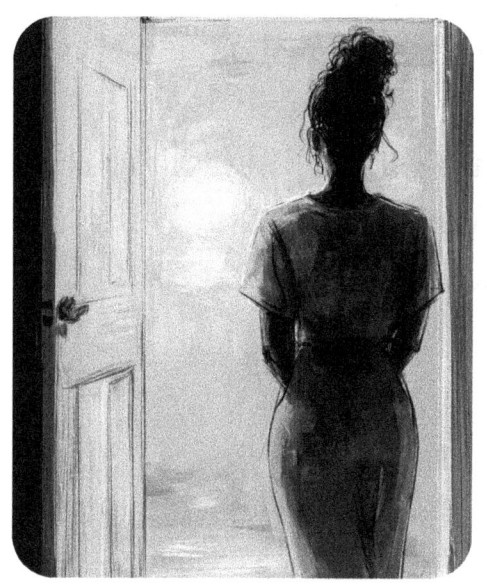

Why you stay is a good question to ask but why you initially got together may be an even better question to determine if the relationship is right for you. What brought you together is often not what will keep you together. You may not even know why you remain in your current relationship or why you stayed so long, but you probably know why you chose to be with your partner.

Call it biological, spiritual, social, or all of the above, the accepted societal norm in traditional relationships is that men be the pursuers. In many cases, men are initially compelled by physical attraction. As such, he will pursue by any means necessary until she either accepts or rejects the pursuit. Even if the object of his desire is unimpressed by him, men are not typically deterred when they are convinced that this person is made for him.

The 1976 Tavares' hit song, "Heaven Must Be Missing an Angel" highlights how a man feels about his new love. While in pursuit, men have been known to spend their last dollar and sacrifice their time to prove that they want to be with that special person. Remember the times on the phone with your partner until the wee hours of the morning, fighting sleep just to hear them breathe? Or traveling hours just to get a glance at your partner, then driving back home without complaint about the time or gas spent?

What changed?! That energy used to "bag" your partner seems to be limited to the initial pursuit. It can't be that there's a communication problem or that one partner lacks the skills to establish an emotional connection because that was often present initially, during the pursuit. In fact, if you go back and look at old love letters, cards, and texts, you may find demonstrated the capacity to emotionally connect with a partner. The answer to "What changed?" is that many people fall into a trap: they pursue winning and not establishing a lifelong connection. After being "bagged," the pursued is left wondering whatever happened to the person that swept them off their feet.

> *Earlier we introduced Ralph and Gwen, the two young, attractive, well-meaning high schoolers. For Ralph the goal was winning Gwen. Success meant letting the world see that he had won her over. The goal for Gwen was a lifelong emotional commitment, wherein love conquered all problems. And we see that eventually that relationship failed. Maybe it was doomed from the start, but both partners had strong reasons to stay.*

Why we stay is an important question to uncover what needs to be done to establish or maintain a healthy relationship. Can you identify positive reasons why you are in your relationship, or are they dwarfed by the many reasons you should leave? Intimate partnerships become stagnant when we only have yesterday's memories. People change over time and what kept the music playing in the beginning of the relationship may not be what keeps us together now. Do you have the same zeal to be together that you had in the beginning? Do you look forward to sharing with your partner about your day? Do you anticipate the new adventures you will have with your partner?

Interest and energy should increase as we progress in the relationship. Imagine what your relationship could be like if you dedicate as much effort now as you did when pursuing your partner. Our job is to continuously build upon the list of "why we stay" rather than hold onto unhealthy reasons. Relationships are choices that we make each day. What have you chosen today?

> ### **Anchors** - *Takeaways*
>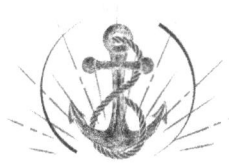
> - Committing is about staying focused on what's mutually important.
> - What brought us together may not be what keeps us together.
> - If fear or domestic abuse is the reason for staying, seek help from local domestic violence agencies/resources!
> - Relationships are choices we make each day.

Excursion 37 - Reasons

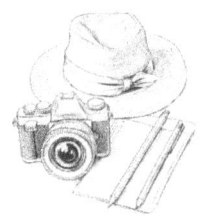

INTRUCTIONS:

Create two lists, one describing why you initially chose to be in a relationship and another of why you remain. If you are no longer in the relationship, then your second list will be why the relationship ended. Prioritize your lists from most important to least important. By prioritizing your lists, you will determine what's driving your choices. After you have constructed both lists, label each item as either H for healthy or U for unhealthy. Evaluate your list and determine which areas need to be addressed.

Initial Reasons   **Current Reasons**

_____   _____

_____   _____

Excursion 38 - Bonus Activity: *Why We Stay Gauge*

INSTRUCTIONS: Reflect on the questions below as you determine what you need to maintain Healthy Me.

- Do you know what you want? (Remember, relationships are not designed to fix you!)

_____

_____

_____

- Do you still see good in your partner? If so, list their good qualities.

　

- Is your partner willing to do the work? If so, what steps have they taken?

　

- What changes do you need to make to establish a healthy relationship?

　

- How do you monitor your progress?

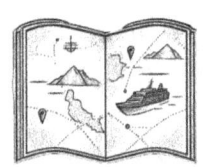 **Charter -** *Bunking Up!*

Many spiritual texts encourage us to do preliminary work before making moves that cement us to one thing or place. One biblical example, Luke 12:28-30, urges us to consider the actual costs before building a house. You may also be familiar with the adage: "Measure twice, cut once!" These messages convey a "first things first" concept.

For a Healthy We , you need to know your and your partner's values and priorities and be clear about how they align. If it's mutually agreeable to take the relationship to the next level, you can then make a commitment to the relationship. Let's use the analogy of flying by plane with an aerial view to survey the land just above your home. This vantage point allows you to see things from a totally different perspective than ground level: You can see how the house sits on the lot and everything that surrounds the house that might enhance or threaten the property.

Having such an aerial view is also important for a relationship because you don't just commit to the individual but rather to everything that comes with that person: children from previous relationships, pets, debts, past trauma, extended family, friends, and the list goes on...

APPENDING – Adding to...
Due to the high incidence of divorce in this country, it's typical to find a partner who has children from a previous relationship. The term blended families describes this family type; the healthiness of these blended families is fast becoming a key indicator for whether their parental relationship will thrive.

Recent data suggests that 66% of marriages involving blending end in divorce. We must therefore pay close attention to this relatively new dynamic to help avoid it adversely impacting your relationship.

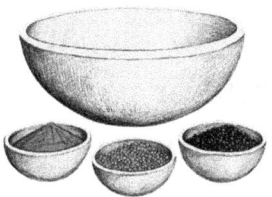

BENDING – Flexing...

The main factor for a successful blending experience is how well the adults (including ex-partners) work together. It's critical that the partners have a clear understanding of each other's role in the system and maintain open communications to avoid creating factions around the child or children. The bottom line is that children follow adults' example. For optimal family dynamics, all adults in the child's life must put the child's best interest ahead of their adult grievances/issues. The adults should therefore agree to neither undermine each other's authority nor speak badly of one another in front of their child. Additionally, the adults must never weaponize the child to harm each other.

AMENDING – Revising & Adapting...

When both partners are blending children from previous relationships, careful assessment and decision-making are needed to identify the best means of introducing the children to each other, along with establishing a process for frequent check-ins, family activities, and discussions. The partners must be open when considering holidays, special occasions, school activities, and vacations. Rather than force the blending, give the children time and space to build relationships with each other. If there is a conflict between blending siblings, all parents (if possible) should be involved to model fairness in problem-resolution.

PENDING – Awaiting Decisions...

The non-biological parent must exercise patience as they form a relationship with their step-child. Remember that the child may see you as an intruder and not a friend. It's important that you are consistent and not impulsive when reacting to the child's behaviors. Also remember to separate the child from the behavior. Don't label the child or place your partner in a position of choosing between you and the child. Once committed to the relationship, your status changed to include the role of blending parent; as such, you must view the child as part of you—more than just a stepchild. Because blending involves more than tolerating the child but embracing this new responsibility, anything short of this will render you detached and compel the child to feel excluded.

RENDING & MENDING – Rips & Repairs

There are so many inherent challenges for blended families that it's not surprising many relationships don't survive the process. The good news is that there are ways to manage this critical aspect of many modern relationships. Because each blending experience is unique and has its own complex variables, there is no definitive prescription for establishing a successful blended family system; but listed below are some guiding principles that will help you with the process:

1. Be realistic about the blending process: a) Don't put too much pressure on yourself; b) Things will probably not go smoothly in the beginning; and c) Blending is a marathon not a sprint. Therefore, if the child's initial reaction isn't favorable, that's okay. Stay positive and stick with it!

2. The non-biological parent must establish their own relationship with the child. Don't depend solely on your

partner to plan activities with the child or to initiate conversations.

3. Be clear about your role in addressing discipline. Most couples defer discipline to the biological parent, but it doesn't mean the non-biological parent sits silently when the child is not following rules. When you speak, focus on what's been agreed upon. Be careful to not go behind the child's back to report wrongdoing to your partner. Address it and be part of the solution.

4. Avoid words like "always" or "never." Give the relationship an opportunity to develop.

5. Support your partner regarding decisions about the child. Remain a united front by not displaying dissension in front of the child.

6. Be prepared to deal with difficult issues that stem from the blending process. In the early stages of the relationship, frequent check-ins and honest discussions are especially critical.

7. Realize the term "step-" has many negative connotations. Be creative in finding healthy ways to describe your new relationship with your partner's child. You are not there to replace the other biological parent, but you ARE a significant adult in the child's life.

8. Don't show favoritism among the children. Be consistent with the rules and decisions for all the children.

9. Blending is not about winning or losing but creating a safe environment to raise healthy children. Don't focus on differences; focus on outcomes. You both are on the same team!

10. Embrace this experience with humility, curiosity, and optimism. Prepare to grow and be pushed outside of your comfort zone. Are you ready for the adventure?

Anchors - *Takeaways*

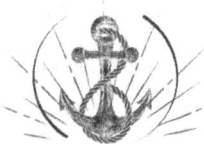

- Blending is a marathon, not a sprint.
- Blending is about creating a safe and healthy environment in which to live and grow.

Excursion 39 - Blended Family Activity:

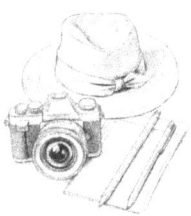

If you are in a blended family, complete the following tasks together:

- Describe the type of blended family you want.

_____
_____
_____

- Develop a plan on how to introduce the children to your partner. Where, when, and how?

_____
_____
_____

- Develop a plan to introduce the children to each other. Where, when, and how?

_____
_____
_____

- Identify the ground rules for blending.

_____
_____

- How will you address discipline for the children? What are the biological and non-biological parents' roles?

_____

_____

_____

- How will you introduce your blended children to others? What phrases/terms will you use?

_____

_____

_____

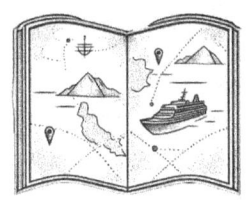 **Charter** - *I Choose YOU*

A recent study titled "Reaching the Modern Independent Woman" found that single women's top three priorities did not include marriage or children. This group instead identified living on their own, establishing a career, and financial security as most important. Many single women have a strong sense of self and reject the traditional stereotype that happiness can only be achieved by marrying and producing offspring.

Until the sexual revolution of the 1960s, society expected young adults to find that special person, wed, and settle down. Although this social norm has lingered into the 21st century, it's less expected as THE norm. More young adults are opting to defer a family for a career. It's now typical to find 30-something adults unmarried, pursuing their passions, and delaying or foregoing marriage and/or parenthood. The American Dream is no longer restricted to the formula of marriage and children and a home in the suburbs. Today the pursuit of happiness looks quite different from the version sanctioned and perpetuated by society and the media.

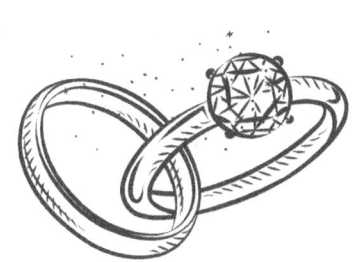

Despite this evolution of expectations, an unchanged fact remains: Choosing to be in a committed relationship is serious business. In addition to realizing what they are signing up for, those who want to pursue a relationship should be mature and self-disciplined to nurture and sustain a healthy relationship.

Earlier in the workbook, we explained that love is a choice. In some cultures, there are arranged marriages; these relationships often work not because of love or compatibility but because of the commitment to cultural expectations. In other cultures, people have the freedom to choose their partners and, unfortunately, many choose for the wrong reasons—attraction being one of those reasons. While attraction may serve to spark the relationship, it can't sustain a relationship over time.

ENVY & JEALOUSY – A Destructive Duo

One of the major challenges in relationships is jealousy, which is rooted in insecurity. Jealousy is experienced when one believes that another is trying to take away something they deem to be solely their own. Jealousy and envy are words frequently used interchangeably despite there being slight differences:

- Envy = I want what you have.
- Jealousy = feeling justified in protecting what I believe to be mine.

Jealousy is an individual problem that our partner cannot solve. For example, we can track our partner's whereabouts or be with our partner around the clock and still experience jealousy. Jealousy stems from a constant need for reassurance; a jealous person needs their partner to repeatedly counter negative messages about themselves or the relationship. A jealous individual exhibits fear of losing someone over whom they have no control.

SIMPLE REMEDY

The most effective way to mitigate jealousy is to simply accept that our partner has chosen us above all others with whom to have a relationship. Anything else will cause us to constantly replay the negative self-talk that boils down to: "Am I good enough for this relationship?" If we are listening to such constant negative self-talk, we should ask ourselves if we are overlaying past negative relationships onto our current partner/situation.

THE Self-cure: Accept that your partner has chosen to be with you and build on that truth.

How do you know when you are ready to make a commitment to a relationship?

- I have established my Healthy Me.
- I am clear about my goals and purpose.

- I have spent time with my partner and understand who I'm selecting.
- Our values and goals are aligned.
- We have clear priorities and are working together.
- We are successful in resolving conflict with each other.
- We enjoy spending time with each other; we know how to have fun.
- We see good in each other and support each other during difficult times.
- My partner accepts all of me: my children, family, career, medical status, etc.
- We have physical and emotional intimacy as well as attraction.

Choosing to be in a relationship is more about you being ready for a commitment than finding the perfect partner. As you've likely already discovered, perfection is an ideal, not reality. Be sure that you commit to Healthy Me before even considering a commitment to Healthy We.

Anchors - *Takeaways*

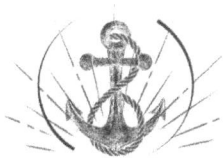

- Attraction can provide the spark of a relationship, but it can't sustain the relationship.
- Envy and jealousy destroy relationships—it is therefore critical to accept that your partner has chosen you so you can manage your self-talk and feelings.
- Choosing to get into a relationship is a declaration of readiness to partner.

Excursion 40 - Envy and Jealousy Activity

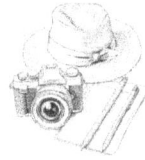

Complete the statements below based on the work you have done in Healthy Me and the time you have spent with your partner.

I choose you because:

_____

_____

_____

I understand who you are, and I have accepted these qualities about you:

_____

_____

_____

I am ready for this commitment because I am healthy and have worked on these areas in my life:

_____

_____

_____

We are entering this commitment based on these mutual values and priorities

_____

_____

_____

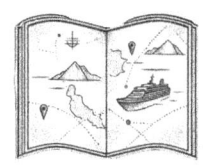 **Charter -** *Commitment to What/Whom?*

Many people think that a commitment to one another forms a healthy relationship. While such dedication is important, the MOST important commitment for a Healthy We is each participant's commitment to a Healthy Me. That's correct: Taking responsibility for, and taking care of, oneself is critical to committing to others.

When we bring our Authentic Self to the relationship each day, our partner can experience consistency and safety. When we commit to Healthy Me, we are committing to truth, love, compassion, giving our best, and seeing good in our partner. Commitment to Healthy Me signals our dedication to our continued growth and development while acknowledging that life may change our perspective but not our core self. It may seem noble to sacrifice ME for the sake of WE—but that is a path for burnout, resentment, and eventual detachment.

"My love for you is so overpowering, I'm afraid that I will disappear."
"Slip Slidin' Away," ~ Paul Simon, 1977

When we commit to bringing our Authentic Self, we can then apply authenticity to our efforts to be a responsible partner. Our actual commitment is NOT to the institution of marriage or other forms of coupling but rather to ourselves and our partner. This means we can still honor our commitment to Healthy We, even if we choose to break up. Because Healthy We means we are compassionate and truthful with one another, it doesn't require that we stay together! We can commit to respectfulness and kindness despite no longer desiring togetherness because we're committing to THE BEHAVIORS. Consider the example of Ralph and Gwen. They grew apart as they got older and eventually decided to divorce. Though initial tensions were high, they exercised their commitment to respectful and kind interactions whenever they encountered one another after they separated.

Many couples mistakenly believe they are demonstrating commitment simply by "hanging on" and losing sight of Healthy Me. But what good is hanging on when Healthy Me is absent and Healthy We is not practiced?

COMMITMENT IS...COMMITMENT IS NOT:

- ...IS far more than what we promise on those special occasions like weddings. It's what we do on an ordinary day, EVERY DAY.
- ...IS NOT merely working hard on a project or behavior but rather dedicating ourselves to bring our truest, best selves.
- ...IS NOT merely being around, but being present and available.
- ...IS recognizing that there is good in the situation and our partner, even when things look bleak.

- ...IS NOT magic, but rather a choice we make each day to embrace our Authentic Self and share it with others.
- ...IS doing what's best for you without intentionally causing harm to others.
- ...IS Healthy Me, which is the <u>mainstay</u> of Healthy We .

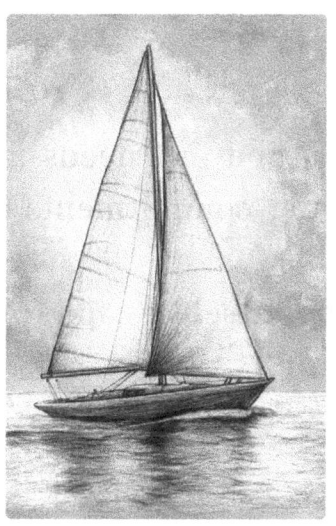

Did You Know? - Stays are a significant part of a sailboat's rigging, and they're essential for safe sailing. Stays support the mast and bear the stress of the wind and the sails. Losing a stay is a serious problem at sea, which is why it's essential to keep your stays in good condition. To have a healthy relationship, we need to do our individual work. Identifying and maintaining the stays in our relationship is an ongoing requirement and critical for a Healthy We .

Making a Healthy We commitment means we understand that we can't change our partner and that each of us must work toward our own Healthy Me. We give ourselves and our partner the space to be authentic.

In 1981, Lionel Ritchie wrote the ballad duet, "Endless Love," which he performed with Diana Ross. The song conveys passion and tenderness as the lyrics suggest that two people become one and pledge their love for each other. How many of us have been to weddings and anniversary celebrations where this famous ballad has been played?

The lyrics suggest that a singular focus on each other begets the titular endless love. But REALationships require much more than passion.

Endless love can only be achieved with the ceaseless work for a Healthy Me : The emphasis is on ME and not the other person. Committing to know ourselves, our wants, and our needs are critical prerequisites for making commitments to others.

> ### **Anchors** - *Takeaways*
>
>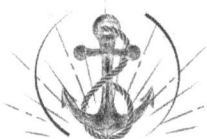
>
> - Knowing ourselves, our wants, and our needs are critical prerequisites for making commitments to others.
> - Commitment means we give ourselves and our partner the space to be authentic.

Excursion 41 - Activity: Healthy Me, Healthy We.

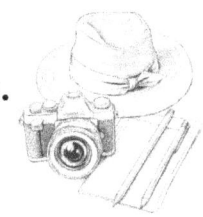

INSTRUCTIONS: Capture your answers below.

1) Identify the steps you have taken to strengthen your Healthy Me.

_____
_____
_____

2) Describe how your Healthy Me has shaped your commitment to Healthy We.

_____
_____
_____

3) Write a mantra that connects your Healthy Me to your commitment to Healthy We.

_____
_____
_____

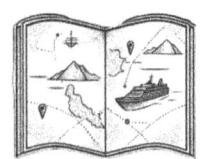

Charter - *Money, Money, Money*

Did you ever wonder why research lists finances as one of the highest-ranking causes of conflict in relationships? Whether it's due to lacking funds, borrowing (and not repaying) funds, or the expectations associated with earning funds, money has been the cause of many a challenge! This charter will spotlight some of these issues, why they tend to linger, and what we can do to avoid running our ship aground.

HOW DID IT BEGIN?

Prior to the Industrial Revolution of the mid-1800s, families produced their own food. Women were actively involved in the daily tasks of farming and raising the children. The Industrial Revolution created a major shift in the U.S. economy because the country transitioned from farm work to factory work, giving women an opportunity to toil outside of the homestead for the first time. Once industrialization took hold, men also left the farm to find work with good wages. Against the backdrop of unequal pay (men earning much higher wages than women), men became the primary breadwinners. This inequity contributed mightily to financial dependency for married and unmarried women alike. During the eras of gender subordination, suffragettes, and gender inequality, societal norms reinforced the notion that men should control how family money was spent.

Since the early 1900s, societal advancements, world wars, and economic developments have contributed to women playing a vital role in every profession, holding jobs from astronaut to zoologist. Women now comprise over 46% of the workforce in America.

WHAT'S THE IMPACT TODAY?

These social shifts have had a major impact on intimate partnerships. Money now represents a major source of conflict for couples. The issues surrounding money vary:

- Some women make more than their partner.
- Some couples struggle with consolidating their financial resources.
- Determining the ultimate decision-maker regarding financial matters is challenging.

Because women attend and complete college at higher rates than men, it's now possible for women to compete with men for higher wage/salary employment. Despite the slowly closing wage-gap between the genders, women are consistently securing more political and economic power. These dynamics have the potential to contribute to a couples' struggle for an appropriate financial balance.

Additionally, our society perpetuates gender-specific roles: We still assume breadwinners are males. As such, men often experience their wife or girlfriend's professional success as an emasculation.

HOW CAN WE OVERCOME MONEY CHALLENGES?

Money is one of those key challenges/choices in relationships that should be addressed before making a commitment to partnership. We must be transparent when our relationship is progressing towards marriage and/or the sharing of financial responsibilities (like the purchase of a home).

While being proactive may seem like more a business merger than an interpersonal partnership, proactivity regarding finances is vital for avoiding future, irreparable damage to the vessel.

Another best practice is to know each other's credit score and understand risk tolerance. Financial goals are just as important as how many children we may desire or where we want to live. The sooner we have these discussions, the more prepared we are for the future.

Lastly, when we set sail as partners, we must remember that we are taking on past and future financial decisions. A rule of thumb for experiencing the smoothest voyage: "Love is sweet, but when the money is funny, our ship can lose its honey!"

Anchors - *Takeaways*

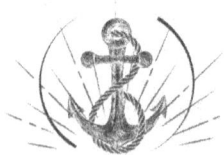

- Money matters.
- Money can represent a major source of conflict for couples.
- Proactivity regarding finances is vital for avoiding future, irreparable damage to your ship.

Excursion 42 - Know Your Score

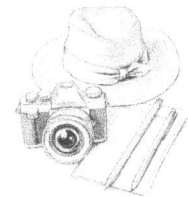

STEP 1: Answer the questions below first for yourself, then for your partner.

STEP 2: Share your results with each other.

STEP 3: Based on the sharing of your results, develop and/or revisit financial goals.

Financial Questions

Myself

1. What did you learn from your family about how to manage your money?
2. Is your risk tolerance low, moderate, or high? Why?
3. What is your credit score, and do you know how to improve your score?
4. Do you have any assets? What did you earn? What was given to you?
5. How much debt do you have? Do you have credit card debt or student loan debt?
6. Do you have an emergency fund?
7. Do you have money in a savings account?
8. What are your financial goals?
9. Do you have a retirement plan?
10. Have you ever filed for bankruptcy and/or do you have any pending financial lawsuits?

My Partner

1. What did they learn from their family about how to manage money?
2. Is your risk tolerance low, moderate, or high? Why?

3. What is their credit score, and do they know how to improve their score?
4. Do they have any assets? What did they earn? What was given to them?
5. How much debt do they have? Do they have credit card debt or student loan debt?
6. Do they have an emergency fund?
7. Do they have money in a savings account?
8. What are their financial goals?
9. Do they have a retirement plan?
10. Have they filed for bankruptcy and/or do they have any pending financial lawsuits?

Healthy We Financial Priorities/Goals

1.

2.

3.

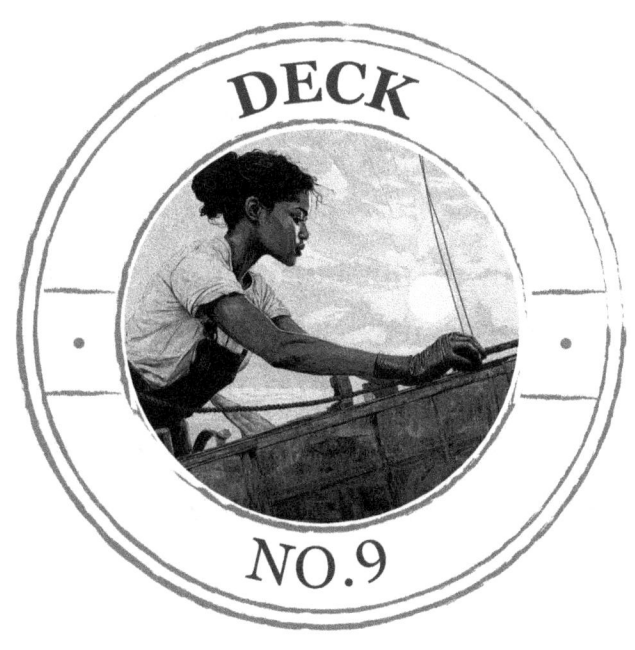

DECK 9

FORTIFY DECK

FORTIFY is the final, though often overlooked, element in bringing our Authentic Self to another's voyage. It's not that we don't intend to fortify and reinforce the relationship, but we often believe our lax and/or subtle methods are adequate. They are not. When we fortify milk, we add nutrients that increase its ability to deliver the health we seek from drinking it. Such is required for REALationships and a Healthy We . Each member must bring their healthiest self possible, then add what is necessary for the ship to remain viable, enjoyable, comfortable, and afloat!

What must be added to a REALationship for it to maintain its viability depends on the vessel. A friendship requires different fortification than an intimate partnership which, in turn, requires distinctly different fortification than a companionship or situationship. Vessels, however, have the same core requirement to remain afloat: crew/members must stay vigilant for threatening environments that could capsize the ship or create barriers to clear communication between crew/members. A vessel maintains its seaworthiness because its crew/members consistently inspect it from stem to stern. When inspections uncover potential problems (or neglected areas that require attention), it's all hands on deck to course correct/make changes.

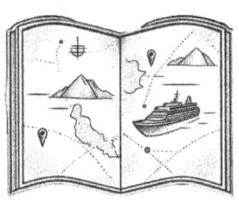 **Charter** - *Getting Unstuck*

What does it mean when an intimate partnership is stuck? Simply put, it's like a ship that has run aground: something should be done about it, or it will eventually lead to a total shipwreck. One common indicator of an intimate partnership being stuck is complaining about the annoyances of the other partner while losing sight of the relationship's benefits.

A recent off-Broadway musical's title provides the quintessential description of the core sentiment for stuck couples: *I Love You, You're Perfect, Now Change!* With these feelings, couples seek counseling because they fail to realize the goal of a REALationship is not to change the other partner. Conflict escalates when we can see the other person's *potential* and we pursue *our need* to expedite *their* change. Most change, however, is not sustainable if there is no personal commitment to that change—no matter how much we love the other person who wants/needs the change to occur. They have to decide to change for themselves.

What can you do if you find that your intimate partnership has run aground? Once again, there are many options, and the best approaches begin and end with YOU. If complaining about the relationship is your primary pastime, try to honestly answer these questions:

- Is my happiness contingent upon my partner making a change?
- If this person makes NO CHANGE AT ALL, will I still feel fulfilled in this relationship?

Guardrails for Getting UNSTUCK

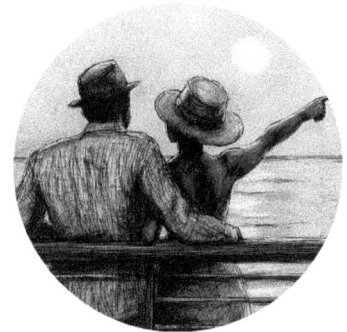

- If your partner is unwilling or resistant to an expressed need for change, this is a set up for conflict, resentment, bitterness, and an eventual shipwreck.

- You must determine the behaviors/habits with which you can live and be happy. Some behaviors will likely need attention to achieve a REALationship.

- The excursion below can help you gain insight regarding what generates the disdain you feel about your partner and the actions you might take. You may find that you've already got the MUST HAVEs, several GAME CHANGERS are in-progress, zero GAME OVER behaviors exist, and holding onto a few INWIs that can finally be tossed out!

Anchors - *Takeaways*

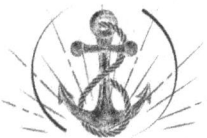

- The goal of a REALationship is not to change the other partner.
- Conflict escalates when we can see the other person's potential and we pursue our need to expedite their change.
- We must determine the behaviors/habits with which we can live and be happy.
- Some behaviors will likely need attention to achieve a REALationship.

Excursion 43 - Activity: INWI

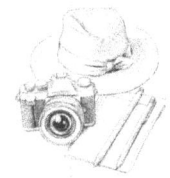

For reference to your responses see Page 258 "Relationshipwrecks"

INSTRUCTIONS: In addition to exploring the guardrails cited above, complete the matrix below. For every insight that results from answering the questions, decide what information you would put into each of the four boxes. To help you, here's the significance of each box and a few examples:

INWI –It's Not Worth It. These are behaviors/habits that, when you honestly explore what annoys you about your partner, are not important enough to expend any additional energy, time, money, or thought. The clearest example of an INWI: Your partner never washes their dishes right away. It's YOUR pet peeve and it's time to let it go.

GAME CHANGER – Annoyances that you've made known to your partner, which they, in turn, are trying to address. You're willing to continue to allow your partner to make the change at their own pace, and you can encourage their progress in a positive manner. An example is smoking cessation: they have made the commitment, are making a concerted effort, may slip-up and smoke but acknowledge the setback, and re-commits their energy to achieving their goal.

GAME OVER – Exactly as implied, these are zero-tolerance behaviors that you are not willing to accept to any degree. Since each of us has different values and tolerance levels, it's difficult to provide the perfect example of a GAME OVER behavior. For some it might be infidelity; for others, possessiveness; and for others still, it may be the seemingly harmless act of leaving the toilet seat up.

MUST HAVE – A staple/critical element that, in its absence, would prevent you from getting or staying involved with a person. For some, a staple/critical element may be spending freedom—the freedom to purchase whatever they can afford without having to provide an accounting to their partner; for others, it might be levity—the uproarious laughter two people can share during an experience. Whatever it is, you know that it feeds your soul and is vital to your wellness in a REALationship. If that which you MUST HAVE dries up, then so, too, would your desire to be in the relationship.

INWI	GAME CHANGER
GAME OVER	**MUST HAVE(s)**

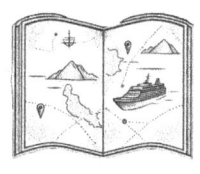 **Charter** - *Sex: It's Good but NOT the Glue of REALationships*

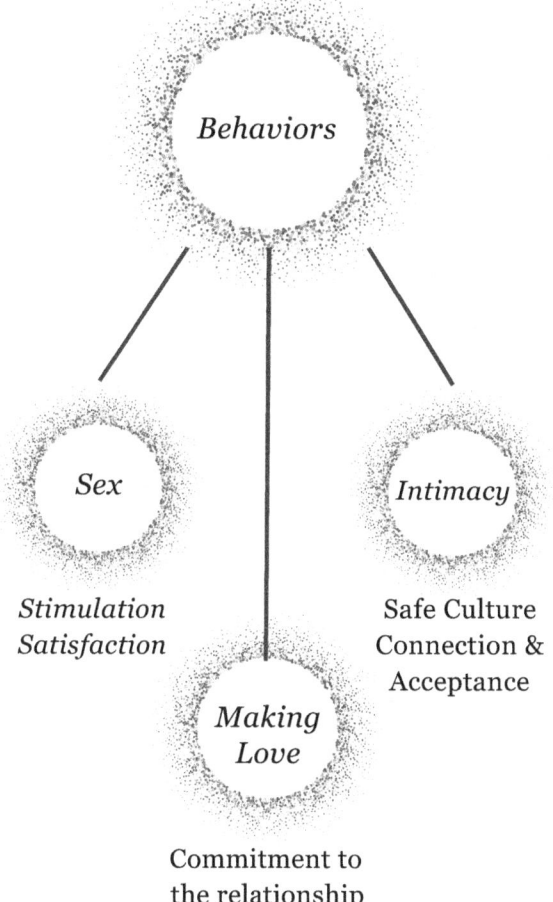

There is a reason this charter occurs toward the end of the workbook: Much is said about sex, but very few people know how to maintain a healthy sex life. Throughout human existence, people have found ways to have sex; after all, sex is natural and only requires attraction and desire. Unfortunately, sex often disappears from the bedroom in long-term relationships, and sometimes rightfully so, when couples aren't on the same page. The truth is there is no expiration date on lovemaking, and sex can remain a part of every committed couple's experience. But how can this goal be achieved?

Let's first distinguish the terms related to sex that often get interchanged due to the physicality involved. Sex, intimacy, and lovemaking differ in their respective objectives and typical impact for those who engage. Sex merely describes a physical experience between one or more individuals that typically involves the stimulation and satisfying of libido/desire. As such, sex can occur without physical intercourse and includes self-pleasure. Intimacy occurs when individuals have created the safe and open culture between one another to express their needs, feel connected, and feel accepted. Lastly, lovemaking is a term reserved for those who have chosen to grow together and maintain their connection via the commitment each has to the relationship. Lovemaking does not always include sex, but sex is often part of the experience.

Benefits of Sex

While sex has the practical purpose of procreation, it also has the power to reinforce the connection between partners or heal and restore a relationship. You've likely heard discussions about making love vs. having sex and wondered: Can we make love without having sex? Can we have sex without making love?

The answer for both questions is yes. Many couples want to make love but find themselves engaging in sex and not fostering their emotional connection. For those couples who seek a connection via their sex or lovemaking, it's important to understand that an emotional connection requires effort. If there is a medical or emotional issue that prevents sexual behavior and results in no emotional connection, a couple should address the barrier to having that connection. If there is a will, there is a way to engage in a healthy and robust sex life.

NOTE: Some people have no desire to have sex and look for partners who are also disinterested in it to create a situation that works for them!

Some Do's and Don'ts Regarding Sex

Frequency - While a healthy sex life is not determined by the quantity of acts, the acts should be frequent enough to keep a spark in the relationship. This means couples must discuss their sexual needs openly and honestly.

Reward & Punishments - Sex is neither a tool nor a weapon. It should never be weaponized or rewarded, but rather sex should be mutual, respectful, and shared as an experience with someone about whom one cares and with whom one feels safe.

Consequences – Because having sex can result in life-changing consequences like unwanted pregnancy, emotional trauma, and sexually transmitted diseases, sex requires that we take care and precautions.

Maintenance - There are many things that can compete with and distract us from the sexual aspects of our committed relationship: children, work, responsibilities, medical challenges, aging, and unresolved conflict in the relationship. While sex can feel liberating and exhilarating, it cannot fix things. Sex is an act that can help solidify an existing connection.

Communication - As a relationship matures, sex should intensify and be more rewarding. For sex to happen, both partners must want it and pursue it. Healthy partners learn to respectfully communicate their needs and accommodate one another. Because our sexual needs and emotional needs change over time, it's critical to avoid settling and instead get busy communicating with one another.

Having sex is a choice to be vulnerable without pretense. There is great cause to celebrate the desire that another human being has for you and all your imperfections. Celebrating means you embrace the opportunity, make adjustments for one another's humanness, and enjoy without judgement.

Anchors - *Takeaways*

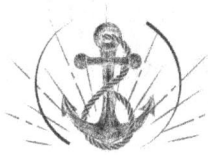

- There is no expiration date on lovemaking, and sex can remain a part of every committed couple's experience.
- Sex has the power to reinforce the connection between partners or heal and restore a relationship.
- As a relationship matures, sex should intensify and be more rewarding.
- For sex to happen, both partners must want it and pursue it.

Excursion 44 - Sex

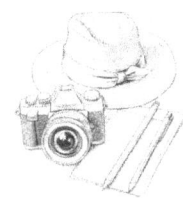

INSTRUCTIONS: Take some time to reflect on these three questions before sharing with your partner. Be prepared to have a deeper discussion that could ensue as a result of your partner's desire to ask these same questions of YOU.

1) What do you consider to be attractive about your partner?

2) What do you know about your partner's needs/desires?

3) What are you willing to expose/be vulnerable about with your partner?

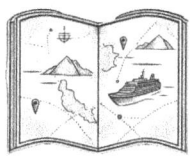 **Charter** - *Intimacy: The Ultimate Relationship*

Reward

As mentioned finding and keeping a Healthy We partner isn't easy. Many relationships start out strong, with each partner participating fully and authentically, but as we grow and age, the components of that once-strong relationship shift, and we risk the eventual severing of the partnership.

The element at the very core of our authentic relationships is intimacy. Intimacy is the glue that can hold us together even as we continue to grow and change. That is the good news; the bad news is that intimacy is often hard to develop and harder to maintain.

Unfortunately, our society often confuses intimacy with sex. While they are both important criteria in a healthy relationship, they are not the same and they are not interchangeable. Sex is a physical activity and while it can lead to or help build intimacy, the depth we can feel and nurture through intimacy is far more rewarding than sex. Because intimacy extends beyond a physical experience, it requires a holistic approach including spiritual, intellectual, emotional, and maybe sexual elements.

When we begin a new relationship, we are cautious about how much to share of our Authentic Self. Authenticity and vulnerability are critical to develop and sustain intimacy, allowing each partner to safely expose who they are. It is that very acceptance of vulnerability where intimacy begins. Without it, intimacy cannot flourish.

Why should we invest the time, effort, and risk to find intimacy in our Healthy We ? For one, intimacy forms a deep companionship that counters and eliminates loneliness. It also improves personal health by reducing stress and releasing positive hormones. It has been documented that intimacy boosts your immune system, lowers blood pressure, and reduces the risk of heart disease.

> *In the movie Dances with Wolves, John Dunbar marries a Sioux woman named Stands with Fist. At one point, he needs to leave the tribe to protect them from harm. He tells his wife that she must remain behind. Her response is not loud, angry, or demanding. She says quietly, "No, we are together as one. I go where you go."*

That is the kind of relationship that can flow out of intimacy.

Do you want to know more about your partner? Is there additional depth to your understanding of your Authentic Self that you have not yet shared?

Do you feel safe within the partnership to learn more about your partner and secure enough to share even more about yourself?

It is never too late to build intimacy in your relationship if both partners are committed to the process. Since the process begins with spending more time together, it may require changes to your schedules and priorities. Perhaps starting a large, collaborative project, or simply expressing what you feel about your partner at the deepest level and encouraging them to do the same can be great starting points. The goal is to get beyond the superficial.

Anchors - *Takeaways*

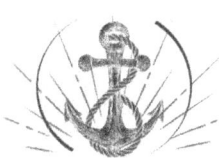

- Authenticity and vulnerability are critical to develop and sustain intimacy.
- Intimacy forms a deep companionship that counters and eliminates loneliness.
- It is never too late to build intimacy in your relationship.

Excursion 45 - Defining Intimacy

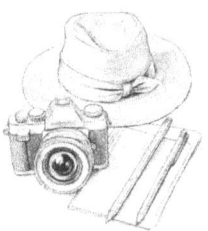

INSTRUCTONS: Discuss with your partner or a close friend how they define intimacy and be prepared to share your own definition.

My definition of intimacy:

_____

Using a 1-5 scale (1=poor; 5= excellent), rate your relationship or friendship's Intimacy Level. Select one partner for this activity and repeat it as often as needed with others.

Intimacy Components: Score

Trust   _____
Acceptance   _____
Physical Affection   _____
Safety   _____
Honesty   _____
Prioritize Quality Time   _____
Express Intimacy Needs   _____
Desire To Know Your Partner/Friend _____
Express Appreciation   _____
Work Together   _____
Total Score   _____

                                   _____

Explanation of Results:

Total Score =

40-50: You are probably comfortable discussing intimacy.

28-39: You may need to venture outside your comfort zone to achieve intimacy.

15-27: This may be a new idea for you. If your partner/friend is also not comfortable, you can use a discussion of the above items as a starting point in the process.

10-14: It may be helpful for you to begin conversations about intimacy with a professional coach, counselor, or therapist who can help you with acceptance.

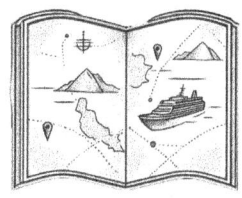

Charter - *Sex is a Privilege, not a Right*

PRIVILEGE – An advantage/access ***granted*** to another.

RIGHT – Legal, social, or ethical entitlement ***owed*** to another.

THE HISTORY OF SEX

Although sex has existed since the beginning of time, people still struggle to understand how to maintain a healthy sex life. Religions and cultural norms have tried to establish rules and structures for this complex aspect of human engagement, but what remains elusive is a clear understanding of sex as an experience and the ground rules for partaking in it.

FROM TABOOS TO PROHIBITIONS

The universal taboo for incest was established and remains for the protection of children and to prohibit family members from compounding and perpetuating genetic birth defects. The protection of children may not have been THE top priority (many cultures considered 12-/13-year-old girls as "ripe" for marriage when the only socially sanctioned sexual intercourse was between married couples). During the Roman Empire, such practices were accepted until they were replaced by the Christian prohibition of sexual experience (for women) unless married. More recently, when the Puritans arrived in America, they imposed strict standards regarding sex. It was limited to married couples, and partaken strictly for procreation and NOT for pleasure.

SEXUAL REVOLUTION(S)!

By the late 1920s, women emancipated themselves from rigid church ideology and began to embrace their sexuality. A likely contributor to this new dynamic was the impact of World War I, which created a demand for women laborers due to the enlistment of men into the military. Their roles outside of the household exposed many women with their first taste of independence, self-reliance, and proof that they could contribute more than offspring and a neat home. Women were trained to do "men's" work and with that came a desire to have similar freedoms and bodily autonomy that, before the war, was much more the exception than the rule for women.

The second sexual revolution occurred in the 1960s-1970s, during which sex was celebrated as an individual choice. Society reduced many barriers to sex and slackened its restrictions for how people could express their sexuality. While we gained many benefits from such advancements, we still wrestle with some of the drawbacks that linger today: Practices like institutionalized sex-trafficking and the rapid expansion of internet pornography.

HOW CAN WE EXPERIENCE THE GOOD WITHOUT PERPETUATING THE BAD?

The 21st century heralded a hook-up culture: Love and intimacy are not requirements to partake in sex, just open-mindedness without judgement. While this may sound simple, people bring their unique desires, expectations, lived experiences (bad and good!), and even past traumas to their sexual relationships—and it is this which creates the need for establishing and understanding the boundaries that render sex a healthy or hurtful experience. Here are some DO's and DON'Ts that can help position us for sexual experiences that are healthy for you and your sexual partner.

DO

- Ensure that the sex is consensual between responsible individuals who understand the benefits and consequences of their choices. A committed relationship does not give any person the right to expect sex on demand. Sex is an experience in which committed couples may choose to engage but are not obligated to provide.
- Limit sex to those who have had a serious conversation about the topic. Sex can have potentially life-changing consequences, and there's a level of responsibility needed to meet one another's needs.
- Quickly address any barriers to openly engaging with your partner so disruption with your connection can be avoided.
- Ensure that sex occurs in a safe space with no preconditions.

DON'T

- Don't use sex to inflict harm on others or to control or manipulate the other person.
- Sexual abuse can and does happen in relationships, including forcing a partner to watch pornography, sabotaging birth control, threatening to cause harm unless sex is given, or threatening to share private information with others.
- Don't weaponize sex to control your partner or seek vengeance for wrongdoing. Infidelity or a lack of trust can cause one or both partners to shut down emotionally and become unavailable for physical intimacy.
- Don't forget each of you is HUMAN. There are various reasons why a relationship runs cold. Sometimes there are medical issues that can impede a couple's sex life and often embarrassment can keep a partner from seeking medical help to remedy the problem. Unresolved trauma can also suffocate the desire for intimacy because triggers remind us of the trauma.

Sex is a beautiful paradox. It can foster a sense of closeness and pleasure, while it can also cause feelings of frustration and isolation. If your goal is a fluid sex life (both parties able to freely give without using coercive control or levying threats), it's critical to engage in sex by applying our healthiest self—our Authentic Self—to remove barriers to a healthy relationship. When we exercise the behaviors outlined in this charter, we position ourselves to experience sex at its very best: as a gift that we give each other.

Anchors - *Takeaways*

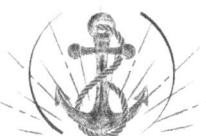

- Healthy couples work through their conflict in a timely manner to avoid lapses in their sex life.
- Ensure that sex occurs in a manner and space that feels safe and without preconditions.
- Barriers to a fluid sex life may include medical issues or trauma. Be kind and willing to explore reasons.

Excursion 46- Reflection Activity

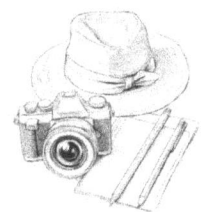

INSTRUCTIONS: Consider the following questions:

- Identify your/their needs and expectations for maintaining a healthy sex life within your relationship.
- If your needs and expectations differ, how will you reconcile the differences?
- Identify barriers that may keep you from engaging in sex with your partner.
- What steps will you take (or have been taken) to assure that you maintain a healthy physical connection with your partner?

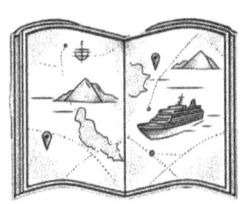 **Charter** - *Keep the Music Playing*

Some say that the true indicator of success is not being able to buy a luxury car, but rather being able to maintain that luxury vehicle! The maintenance of any car can be expensive, and a luxury vehicle's maintenance is even more costly. The same can be said about quality relationships: establishing the relationship may be the first success, but fortifying the relationship is the ultimate achievement. Keep in mind that longevity alone is not necessarily an indicator of relationship health. We mentioned earlier in the workbook that people stay together for many reasons, and some reasons have little to do with love.

Fortify: to protect, strengthen, bolster, support

When we value something, we take measures to protect it. When we value our relationship, we demonstrate it by investing in the other person or situation. What does investing in another person look like? For starters, we demonstrate that we're invested by being proactive in preserving the relationship: we anticipate there will be differences, and we make time to discuss these as much as we can (see Share, Align) so we're not blindsided by them when they surface. Yet Fortifying does NOT mean that we seek to dominate or restrain, but rather to treasure.

Consider the many things we fortify because we seek to enhance their value and impact in our lives:

FOOD – cereals, breads, drinks. The next time you shop for groceries, take notice of the many labels that indicate how the product's nutritional value is increased due to FORTIFICATION.

STRUCTURES – As you drive around, notice the fortification of roads, bridges, building foundations, and levees. Anything that experiences wear & tear requires strengthening over time. Despite the very best architectural blueprints and materials, time and usage necessitate fortification!

MILITARY SCIENCE – All branches of service use permanent and field fortifications to strengthen positions that could be vulnerable to ambush or attack. Elaborate forts and troop shelters are erected in times of peace and when there is threat of war.

An earlier excursion in the Pursue deck explored the practice of spending quality time together and pursuing mutual priorities. Such pursuits should also include identifying ways to stay connected to each other. Additionally, borrow from the example of the military: expect challenges, even if the relationship is healthy. Discuss and plan for how to manage conflict so an approach is available when conflict inevitably occurs!

Lastly, the goal is for us to nurture relationships beyond intimacy. In the 1982 rom-com Best Friends, two writers, after dating for five years, decide to marry. The couple takes a train ride from the west coast to the east so they can meet their respective in-laws and inform them of their marriage. Comedy ensues as they struggle with changes in their relationship dynamics once they've made the commitment to marry. "How Do You Keep the Music Playing?" is an Oscar-nominated duet from the Best Friends soundtrack, sung by James Ingram and Patti Austin. The lyrics highlight the embedded challenges of fortifying a relationship while maintaining our core friendship and Authentic Self.

Let's visit some of the important questions associated with maintaining our Authentic Self while committing to journey through life with another person:

Question: *How do we maintain the good aspects of our relationship?*

1. Answer: Healthy relationships are an ongoing JOURNEY and not a vacation from reality. As happens while journeying, expect there to be good times, responsibilities, setbacks, and surprises.

Question: *How will we know our relationship is healthy?*

2. Answer: Healthy individuals embrace one another's Authentic Self.

Question: *How can we keep our relationship "fresh?"*

3. Answer: Healthy individuals create an ongoing practice of Exploring, Accepting, Healing, Growing; bringing that attitude to their relationships.

Dilemma: *What if it feels like our love is slipping away?*

4. Healthy individuals acknowledge that love is a choice.

Dilemma: *What if the changes in our relationship seem to affect the status of our relationship?*

5. Answer: Healthy relationships are continuously GROWING.

Fortifying is INTENTIONAL. Avoid embracing the countless lyrics that suggest love alone will conquer all! The reality is that each partner must commit to self-development and managing the changes that their lives present.

It's also important to accept that we can never connect with our partner the same way we did when we first met. We must spend time together; sharing with one another far beyond the Commit deck. If dialogue stops, we cannot know our partner. We must, therefore, not only work to preserve our relationship but also strengthen and enhance it through connection and curiosity.

Anchors - *Takeaways*

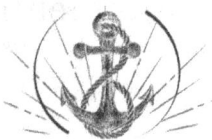

- When we value our relationship, we demonstrate it by investing in the other person.
- Healthy relationships are an ongoing journey.
- Healthy individuals expect and accept that their partners will change over time.

Excursion 47- Develop a Fortification Plan

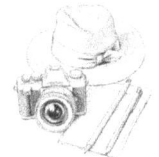

Since Healthy We promotes proactive behaviors, developing a **Fortification Plan** is critical. This plan provides a framework for maintaining healthy behaviors for keeping the music playing. Your Fortification Plan should be fluid, providing the opportunity to make changes as needed.

INSTRUCTIONS: Create your fortification plan

My/Our Fortification Plan

1. **Connect.** Establish several ways to stay connected with your partner.

2. **Share.** Establish formal and informal communication paths. Ensure that you identify a frequency for communicating that is mutually amenable.

3. **Self-Development.** Identify ways you intend to continuously grow.

4. **Compassion.** What specific efforts do you make to see/acknowledge the good in your partner, especially when things are not good?

FROM THE BRIDGE - ADDITIONAL RESOURCES & REFERENCES

A ship's bridge is where the captain can see what's happening and issue commands. In this section of the book, we provide the complete Healthy Me, Healthy We illustrated model to help you envision aspects of REALationships discussed in earlier decks. Regardless of your desired destination, a view from the bridge represents the big picture of your journey for a Healthy Me and a Healthy We .

Healthy Me, Healthy We - The REALationship Model

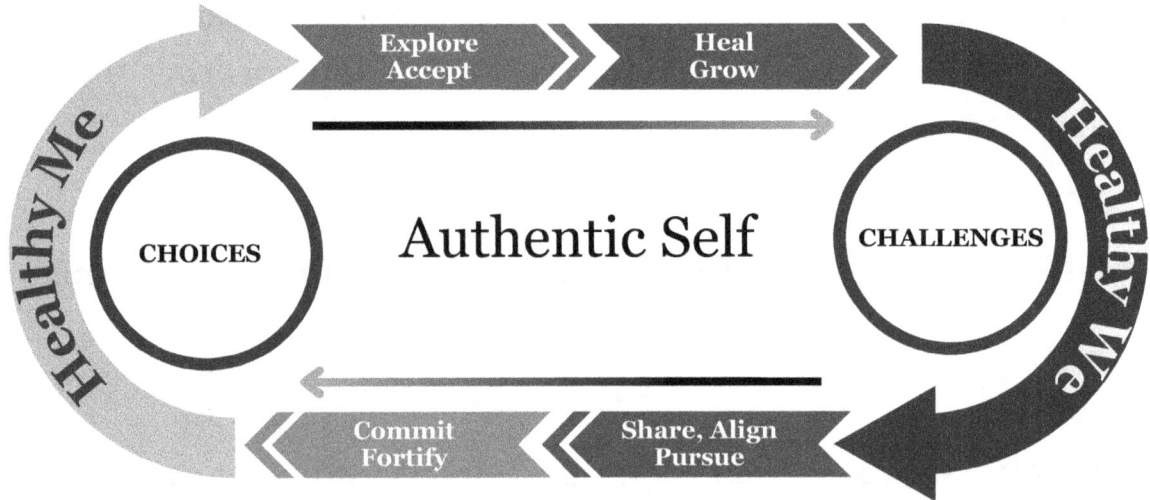

The HMHW model considers human nature—the toggle between managing personal needs/issues as we contribute to the dynamics of interpersonal relationships. To that end, the HMHW model is fluid to reflect reality: Life's challenges and choices don't present themselves in a linear fashion but randomly. Additionally, the HMHW model has an elliptical shape and its components are contrasting chevrons to suggest motion—as if on a track—

clockwise and counter-clockwise, respectively. These tracks suggest human tendency; be it as an individual or interpersonal, our emotions are ever-flowing and ceaseless, like the dynamo whose parts work to create energy.

And finally, we call the HMHW model a REALationship model. It incorporates the reality of working toward achieving healthiness and therefore, healthy REALationships versus facades based on platitudes. It's critical for individuals to understand—much like being in a large theme park—where in the model they are, and at any given point of development—as they work toward Authentic Self and healthy REALationships.

Some see our HMHW model and ask, "Where is the component that represents dysfunction?" To that question, we offer this simple explanation: there is dysfunction in every human dynamic because people are NOT perfect. For that reason, we chose to eliminate dysfunction as a distinct component and rather assume that each person has their own dysfunction—providing their own distinguishing brand for an otherwise universal, human characteristic. This is not meant to be critical but merely to point out that each of us brings some degree of dysfunction-to-be-managed to every relationship—even if we choose to live alone on a deserted island. Dysfunction is just another way of saying "human."

Here's an overview of each component of the HMHW model, the way it can be experienced in real time. To simplify our explanations and examples, we'll use an intimate couple as our frame of reference.

Many couples find that though they may have started their relationship on what felt like a good note, it devolved from the honeymoon into a dynamic of unhealthy interaction patterns and unsuccessful attempts at healthy conflict resolution. Over time, many couples develop unhealthy habits for dealing with the inevitable conflicts that arise in relationships. Their issues become compounded by the ways they either avoid the conflict or their ineffective methods for addressing conflict. They may even seek help to improve the quality of their relationship, but all too often, by the time the couple engages in professional help, deep scars have likely developed—scars that act as a barrier to moving forward. We'll use this typical dynamic to clarify some of the examples of the HMHW model.

Healthy Me has three components:

- Explore
- Heal/Accept
- Grow

The actions pursued in these components bring us to our Authentic Self. This Authentic Self is not about perfection, but instead suggests that we embrace who we are and that we are comfortable with our total package. What's more, identifying our Authentic Self means that we know our strengths and challenges, and that we are working towards our purpose. Our Authentic Self allows us to have inner peace, a peace that eliminates our search for people and things to fulfill us. When we are authentic, we are complete and accept that we are unique and we have something special to offer others.

Challenges and Choices

"Being challenged in life is inevitable. Being defeated is optional."
~Roger Crawford

This quote by Hall of Fame motivational speaker and author Roger Crawford reinforces the components of the HMHW REALationships Model. EVERYONE faces challenging situations. Since it's impossible to navigate life without experiencing difficulties, setbacks, disappointments, and the like, the most effective preparation is to accept their inevitability and learn from each challenge we face. For this reason, our model references these challenges to remind us that something always stands between our goals and successful achievement: animal or mineral, normal or paranormal, clearly visible or invisible. Whatever the obstacles, one of the most important provisions we can carry with us is our attitude, a mindset that helps us absorbs life's storms and headwinds.

If we accept and anticipate that our journey through life will be fraught with challenges, the attitude that most helps us to prepare and prevail is represented by the second circle in the HMHW model: choices. None of us can control the future or the adversity the future may hold for us; however, we can control the mindset we apply when adversity visits or is looming on our horizon. When we choose our attitude, we place ourselves in a better position for successfully navigating whatever challenges beset us.

In this way, the HMHW model reminds us that our journey to our Authentic Self is not a once-and-done trip through Explore/Accept/Heal/Grow, respectively, but rather many excursions with countless challenges and endless decision-points. That is life. To partake in its healthiest journey, we each must face the challenges and own our choices and their impact.

Healthy We has two main components: Share/Align/Pursue, and Commit/Fortify.

These components complement the Healthy Me who is authentic. The actions pursued in these components allow for the healthiest relationships, or what we describe as a REALationship. A REALationship suggests that each person is doing their best to bring their Authentic Self as described in the Healthy Me sections to the relationship. REALationships (like individuals) do not suggest perfection or a match made in heaven, but instead means that each of us is doing our own work and bringing the most authentic person to others. Remember our Authentic Self allows us to have inner peace, a peace that eliminates our search for people and things to fulfill us. When we are authentic, we are complete and accept that we are unique and have something special to offer others. That something special is our contribution to each aspect of the relationships in which we engage.

This happens through five actions we must take:
- Share
- Align
- Pursue
- Commit
- Fortify

SHARE is where friends, couples, companions, etc., begin. When we involve ourselves with others, we share who we are, our values, and vision for our life. This includes our flaws and foibles. Our strengths, lessons learned, and individual needs are all part of the invitation we extend to the trusted other and hope that they will accept whatever challenges they may encounter during the voyage, our REALationship. There is NO substitute for sharing. If you use the excuse of not having time, what you're saying is, "I don't have the time to sustain what we found." It's also wise to share your barnacles. Being vulnerable is good for REALationships.

ALIGN Upon receiving what is shared, each of us has a choice to sign onto the journey or not. If the desire is mutual, it's critical for each of us to determine the many ways we are a good fit for one another, where there is need for enhancement, and where the differences exist but don't matter enough to address. The more aligning we do, the better foundation we establish for Pursue/Commit/Fortify.

PURSUE There will always be differences in our outlooks, skills, priorities, backgrounds, and countless other facets—none of us are clones, nor must we be. What's most important is for us to maintain our Authentic Selves as we journey together.

For ours to be a successful, happy, healthy voyage, we must have common pursuits in addition to our personal/individual pursuits. It's not enough to be aware of ways we align; we must ensure that we're chasing what we both determined to be important. If only one of us is doing all the work, the likelihood of a shipwreck is high.

COMMIT may sound simple and straightforward, but it's often one of the most difficult endeavors to maintain. None of us is the exact same person we were just yesterday, and slight changes, over time, can produce a kind of veering off course that can happen. Think about how easily gaining just one or two pounds per month can impact your entire wardrobe! The key of Commit is to stay focused on what was mutually determined to be important. Revisit those priorities and original mindsets to ensure the engagement levels are still mutually high. Apply the adage: "We can never step into the same river twice" as a reminder that everything changes and so do the priorities we established when we first embarked. Commit means being intentional about revisiting and, if necessary, reestablishing priorities throughout the voyage.

FORTIFY is when we bring our Authentic Self to one other's voyage. It's not that we don't intend to fortify and reinforce the relationship, but we often believe our lax and/or subtle methods are adequate. They are not. When we fortify milk, we add nutrients that increase its ability to deliver the health we seek from drinking it. Such is required for REALationships, or a Healthy We . Each member must bring the healthiest individual possible then add what is necessary for the ship to remain viable, enjoyable, comfortable, and afloat!

What must be added to a REALationship for it to maintain its viability depends on the vessel. A friendship requires different fortification than an intimate partnership which, in turn, requires distinctly different fortification than a companionship or situationship. Vessels, however, have the same core requirement to remain afloat: crew/members must stay vigilant for threatening environments that could capsize the ship or create barriers to clear communication between crew/members. A vessel maintains its seaworthiness because its crew/members consistently inspect it from stem to stern! When inspections uncover potential problems (or neglected areas that require attention), it's all hands on deck to course correct/make changes.

CAPTAINS' LOG

"I don't need YOU to love me..."

~ *"I'm Here," The Color Purple*

Each day we live means there is hope for improvement in our lives and relationships. Loving ourselves is the key to allowing others to love us—be they friends, companions, intimate partners, or a combination of all three. The foundation for healthy love is to know and bring our Authentic Self to everything. This means we're doing our individual work, which in turn means we're addressing our own needs and NOT relying on others to fill our needs. This ongoing pursuit frees us to enjoy a relationship without encumbering each other with the burden of completing the other person.

It's a continuous loop. Find You. Be You. Bring You – to all that you do alone or with others. That's what makes it a REALationship.

Charles Frazier's Final Thoughts: It's never too late...to discover and embrace Healthy Me!

"The two most important days in your life are the day you were born and the day you find out why." -Mark Twain

This workbook was written to empower every individual to seek and achieve a Healthy Me. Despite all of us being born with specific gifts, abilities, and our own unique purpose, many of us don't discover that truth until our later years. As infants and toddlers, we didn't even consider the concepts "I can't" or "It's too hard;" instead we imagined there was NOTHING beyond our abilities. As time passed, however, we learned to limit ourselves. Although life experiences are designed to help us develop and mature, these experiences also can act as barriers to our growth and development. Additionally, many of us have unresolved traumas that have impeded our journey to a Healthy Me. Despsite that, it's not too late to become the best YOU!

If we live long enough, we all experience some form of trauma. Realizing and acknowledging what's in our life baggage is critical. Yet so many go through life never unpacking our baggage. We instead tend to tuck our life baggage away somewhere, rendering it hidden from others—and ourselves. Many of us seek out relationships to help us feel completed and/or as though what we've hidden will remain stuffed away. Relationships don't create additional content for our baggage; they reveal what's in our life baggage and expose unresolved emotional wounds. But there is good news: We can still be healthy with a tarnished past IF we are willing to do our own work.

Our work cannot be substituted by avoidance, projection, manipulation, addiction, or distraction. Healthy Me means we own who we are and accept every experience as a means of getting closer to our Authentic Self.

While each of us is born with a purpose and gifts, over time, our purpose and gifts can evolve to become clearer to ourselves and others. When we embrace our Authentic Self and present a Healthy Me, we don't compare ourselves with others but instead embrace our uniqueness unapologetically.

For those who invest the time to work through Healthy Me —the first part of this workbook—the rewards include more confidence and peace of mind, but not perfection. Despite those mistakes, your Authentic Self/Healthy Me is equipped to acknowledge shortcomings and learn from your experiences.

With that said, Authentic Self/Healthy Me is dynamic because we are always confronted with life challenges and choices. So, we must keep nurturing our Authentic Self/Healthy Me through our self-care and accountability plans. A self-care plan consists of:

a) Regular activities we do to take care of our holistic self, and
b) A few people in our inner circle with whom we can be REAL (who can give us the feedback we need rather than what we want them to say).

Remember: Without Healthy Me, it's difficult to find and sustain our Authentic Self. Loving ourselves should be joyful. Start loving and taking care of YOU!

SELF-CARE Activity

Develop a self-care plan that allows you to nurture your Authentic Self/Healthy Me. Listed below is an outline you can modify to fit your needs. The Self-Care Plan can/should change over time as you learn more about you and your needs.

Self-Care Plan

1. Self-Regulating Activity: ways to manage your emotions. (i.e., yoga, meditation)
2. Physical Activity: hiking, swimming, biking, etc.
3. Fun: What makes you smile and feel happy (whether done alone or with others)
4. Self-Development: Areas for personal growth.

Accountability Plan

Identify two to three people in your inner circle who you trust to be accessible and who'll give you constructive feedback. Formally ask these individuals to:

a) Be part of your Accountability Plan and,
b) Check-in with them (even if things are going well.) *

*NOTE: The frequency of the checking in is at your discretion; however, the more you share, the better you will feel.

Cheryl Grayson's Final Thoughts - Stop Blaming and Start Owning

"What I know about me is much more important than what others THINK about me." ~ Cheryl Grayson

Developing these materials for others gave me a tremendous opportunity to look inside myself. From introspecting, I have emerged with an ability to recognize a key to my personal healing and growth which I hope you've absorbed: STOP BLAMING AND START OWNING.

A significant revelation from examining myself and my choices is how I define happiness. I've learned that being happy means being healthy—from the inside out—and nobody except me can make me healthy inside. I am the only person who can define happy for ME. It's no other person's responsibility and nobody else is to blame if I stop pursuing the healthiest, most authentic me. Hence my quote at the very top of the page: I know me and I've learned to make choices based on what's healthy for me rather than what pleases others.

While it took nearly a lifetime for me to learn the above, I want to help others learn it faster: *Healthy Me is the source of happy me and happy me is only possible when I am true to my Authentic Self.* Truth can never erase my past traumas or errors, but understanding myself allows me to live my life with more intention and aligned with what is healthy for me.

Welcome to the journey to discover authentic you and healthy relationships:

"Now voyager, sail thou forth to seek and find." ~ Walt Whitman

STOP BLAMING/START OWNING Activity

The 1988 chart-topping song "Man in the Mirror," is an incredibly catchy tune that helps us remember we must confront ourselves, we can better our situations, and it begins with OURSELVES. While the practice sounds simple, it's probably one of the most under-used approaches. Look into the mirror, see yourself, then ask yourself: What am I contributing to the status quo/change I need?

Part of the difficulty comes from the habit of pointing at ALL the external factors which may, indeed, be contributing. But here's a way I've broken free from the habit of BLAMING to address what I OWN in situations.

INSTRUCTIONS:

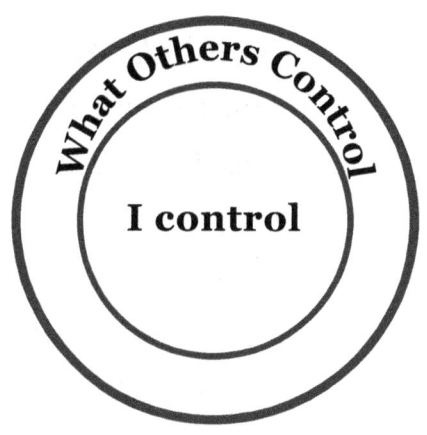

STEP 1: Start with the circle-in-circle illustrated.
Think about three situations you'd like to improve.
For each situation, decide whether it's something you can control or others control. Place each in their respective circle (either you control or others control).

STEP 2: For each situation that others control, remove your immediate focus. (This means let it go and stop dwelling on it for now. You may decide to discuss it with those who control it, but you needn't address it right now.)

STEP 3: For each situation you control, ask yourself the following question(s):

    a) What role am I playing in keeping this going?
    b) Why am I choosing to play that role?
    c) What can I do to change my role?
    d) What is holding me back from doing what I can do?
    e) What is 1 behavior I can change that will break my pattern of holding myself back?

STEP 4: DECIDE. Does the situation you're committing to address require discussion with others? (e.g., Will they be impacted by a change in your pattern of behavior?)

If the answer is YES, share your intentions/new approach with those stakeholders who will experience a different behavior from you by:

Establish Alignment regarding one another's plans for dealing with the new approach, in the most positive way possible. (e.g., If others will experience you being less dependent on their opinion about how you participate in family functions, establish alignment regarding what feels supportive when you attend family functions but participate in a different manner).

Now celebrate! You have taken the initial steps for building a habit of OWNING your contributions to your situation while establishing a foundation for sustaining that new behavior!

Wilbur Pike's Final Thoughts: Listen to the stories around you and let them influence Authentic You

First, I was delighted and humbled to be invited by Charles and Cheryl to help author this book. The topic has long been a source of interest for me as I continue to learn who I really am and embrace what I find.

So, the position of all three authors is that we are no more perfect than any of the readers of this book. Perhaps we do have a gift to offer in that the discovery and development of Authentic Me and the possible Authentic We has been a lifelong study for the authors. In this book we share what we have learned thus far, but the voyage is never over and we reserve the right to be in development, just like our readers.

I am a storyteller. Since childhood, I have been captivated by the idea that the overwhelming learning reality for humans is verbal. If we view human development historically, most of our time on earth has been spent in education through the spoken word. For Indigenous Americans, for example, before the European influx, virtually every bit of the education of youth came through stories. By hearing those stories and imagining oneself within them, the legends of their society became the classroom and the history for an entire population.

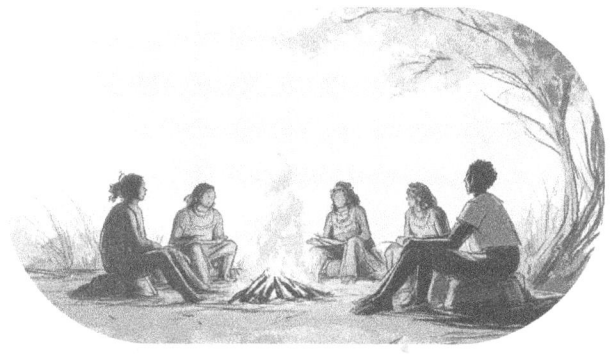

My stories flow from my experiences or my imagination of experiences I have yet to have. I reserve the right to alter a story that is often repeated. I do so to amplify the messages in the story. My characters are often based on real people I have known in places I have actually been.

Invariably, the morals, ethics and history within storytelling are loud and clear. This has always been a pathway to understanding and accepting my quest for Authentic Self. I am honored to have been able to contribute my stories to this book. As always, the storyteller learns the lessons too.

REFLECTION ACTIVITY

Think of and remember the stories told to you in your youth. No matter how often they were repeated, play them again in your mental theatre and extract the lessons within them.

List below some of the lessons you have derived from the stories.

_____

_____

_____

How have those lessons contributed to your awareness of Authentic You?

_____

_____

_____

www.ingramcontent.com/pod-product-compliance
Lightning Source LLC
Chambersburg PA
CBHW080331170426
43194CB00014B/2529